THE COMPLETE BOOK OF CHILD

CW00322247

Dr B. Robert Feldman is Assistant Attending Physician, Division
of Pediatric Allergy, Columbia-Presbyterian Medical Center, and
Assistant Professor of Clinical Pediatrics at Columbia College of
Physicians and Surgeons, both in New York City.

David Carroll is the author of more than a dozen books, including
The Complete Book of Natural Medicines.

B. ROBERT FELDMAN, MD WITH DAVID CARROLL

The Complete Book of *Children's Allergies*

PAN BOOKS LONDON, SYDNEY AND AUCKLAND

First published in the USA by Times Books, a division of Random House,
Inc., New York, and simultaneously in Canada by Random House of
Canada Ltd, Toronto

This edition first published in Great Britain 1988 by Pan Books Ltd
Cavaye Place London SW10 9PG

9 8 7 6 5 4 3 2 1

ISBN 0 330 30156 X

Phototypeset by Input Typesetting Ltd., London SW19 8DR
Printed in Great Britain by Richard Clay (The Chaucer Press) Ltd.,
Bungay, Suffolk

To my wife, Clare, who provided constant encouragement, my children David and Janet who knew that eventually it would be completed, and finally in loving memory of my parents: Morris and Florence Feldman.

—B.R.F.

Contents

Acknowledgements

First, let me acknowledge the unknowing contribution of all the patients I have cared for during the past twenty-two years. Their constant questions provided me with the incentive to think about and eventually to write this book.

My sincere appreciation to my close friend and colleague, William J. Davis, MD, director of the Allergy Division, Babies Hospital, Columbia-Presbyterian Medical Center, and to my long-time associate, Charles H. Feldman, MD, for reviewing the manuscript and providing me with their constructive criticism.

Finally, to my co-author, David Carroll, who with his literary talent has left his indelible imprint on this book, I extend my thanks for a difficult job well done.

—B.R.F.

Part One

An Introduction to Allergy

CHAPTER ONE

About Allergy

It is estimated that approximately 15 to 20 per cent of the population suffer from some kind of allergic condition. Many of your friends are no doubt numbered among them, and if you are a member of this not-so-exclusive club your child probably is too, for allergic tendencies can be inherited. But first things first.

If your child is an allergy sufferer, you already know all you care to concerning the symptoms this difficult malady brings: the sneezing, the wheezing, the all-night bouts with the vaporizer. There is, however, an invisible mechanism that works behind these outward signs which is little understood even by many long-time allergy sufferers. Let us examine what triggers this common, familiar, yet basically mysterious quirk of the human machine.

WHAT IS AN ALLERGY?

There are many ways to define allergy, most of them unduly technical. For our purposes an allergy is simply an abnormal response of the body to a substance that is ordinarily harmless for most people. Grass pollens are a good case in point. Invite ten of your friends on a picnic; let them settle down to enjoy the spread. The majority will probably be quite happy, but the chances are that one or two will find that exposure to grass pollens will bring on unpleasant symptoms in the nose and eyes. The nose itches and produces sneezing and the eyes stream. The meaning of this is that most people exposed to grass pollens will not react at all but those of us who are allergic to these substances can, and will, exhibit a variety of symptoms.

The skin, nose and lungs are the parts of the body most commonly involved during an allergic episode – the section of the body where the allergic attack takes place is called the shock organ – though the list of organs which may possibly come under siege does not stop here. It includes:

the nose (hay fever)

the lungs (asthma)

the skin (rashes)

the eyes (allergic conjunctivitis)

the stomach (food sensitivities)

the ears (fluid behind the eardrum)

the head (headaches and sinus troubles)

Allergic symptoms may involve a single part of the body: the lungs in asthma or the skin in atopic dermatitis. In some conditions such as hay fever the eyes and nose will be involved, and in anaphylaxis, which is a generalized form of allergic reaction, the lungs, skin, central nervous system, and heart will take part in the response.

ALLERGENS AND ANTIBODIES

When does an allergic reaction begin? Basically, it starts the moment a child comes in contact with a foreign substance known as an allergen or antigen (though not exactly synonymous, the two terms are often used interchangeably), and becomes sensitized to this allergen. Antigens are foreign substances (proteins and poly-saccharides) that can cause an immune response in any person. An allergen is a type of antigen that is capable of causing symptoms in an allergic individual.

We will take a closer look at the allergic mechanism in a following section, but at this point it is necessary only to know that for a sensitized person, allergens are the triggers of allergic episodes, and that they include an incredibly wide spectrum of possible substances ranging from apples to zucchini (courgettes).

The most common offenders include pollen from trees, grasses and weeds as well as mould, dust, foods, industrial pollutants, animal dander, insect stings, and household chemicals such as detergents or perfumes. The most frequent allergies plaguing children are hay fever and bronchial asthma, followed by skin conditions such as hives or atopic dermatitis, sensitivities to such common foods as nuts or dairy products, and reactions to stinging insects.

It is interesting to realize that different children who are sensitive to the same allergen may respond to this substance with totally different clinical symptoms. Whereas five-year-old Brian develops a runny nose and streaming eyes during the pollen season, nine-year-old Alice wheezes whenever she is exposed to this common substance. Why such varying organ-system involvement occurs in reaction to the same allergen is not clearly understood.

Potential allergy-causing substances are thus in our environment every hour of the night and day, whether we are aware of them or not. They enter the human system via four main 'doors':

In the substances we eat: these are called ingestants. Almost any food or drug you can think of may be included, along with an ever-growing number of chemical compounds added to our foods.

In the materials we touch: these are called contactants. Primulas are a prime example.

In the chemicals injected into our bodies: injected materials. These include medicines such as penicillin and insulin.

In substances we inhale: inhalants. While pollen grains are the most common offenders, industrial and household pollutants are enemies to be reckoned with.

Most children will not develop signs or symptoms of allergy regardless of the number of allergens to which they are exposed. However, for approximately 10 to 20 per cent of children in the UK, and as many as 1 in 3 children in Australia and New Zealand, contact with these otherwise harmless allergens will trigger an allergic response. We do not know why one child develops this type of reaction and a sibling or the child next door fails to do so. Nevertheless, we do have the answers for many of the questions asked about why allergies begin.

IT'S IN YOUR GENES

We know, for example, that when a child's parents or grandparents are allergic, the chances of that child developing allergic symptoms are greater than those of a child born to a nonallergic family. On a statistical basis, though exact numbers are difficult to obtain, approximately 10 to 20 per cent of all children will develop some kind of allergic problem. Those youngsters with one allergic parent will have about a 30 to 35 per cent chance of joining the ranks of the allergic, and if both parents are allergic, the possibility jumps to 50 or 60 per cent, more than one in two. If there is absolutely no history of allergy in a child's background, he or she still has about a one in six chance of developing an allergy. So the end result is that while a family history of sensitivity is usually but not *inevitably* a ticket to allergy, a lack of it in the family background does not guarantee immunity.

While there is a strong genetic tendency towards allergy among certain children, *specific sensitivities* are not inherited. It is the *potential* to develop allergy that is passed on from parent to child, not a particular allergic condition.

Take, for example, a young mother named Elizabeth who is sensitive to dogs and cats. Her son Stephen is also born with allergies, but his attacks are set off by grass. Another mother, Valerie, has two children, a boy and a girl. Both are allergic, but their reactions differ not only from each other's but also from their mother's. Valerie's son sneezes when he is exposed to feathers, and her daughter develops a rash whenever she drinks milk. Valerie herself has asthma. Moreover, even if a parent has an especially severe allergy, the children will not necessarily develop either this particular allergy *or* its particular intensity – neither specific sensitivity nor degree of seriousness is inherited.

AT WHAT AGE DO ALLERGIC SYMPTOMS USUALLY DEVELOP?

The time it takes for a person to become sensitized to a specific allergen can vary from months to decades. Why is it that a person can be exposed over and over again for many years to the same allergen and then on a certain hour of a certain day, seemingly out of the blue, have a reaction to it? No one knows. But this is how the process works. The common notion that if you did not have hay fever as a child you will never get it as an adult is a myth.

I know, for example, of one twenty-nine-year-old woman who rarely sneezed. On a cross-country driving trip she and her husband stopped to camp somewhere in the deserts of New Mexico, a region to which, ironically, many with allergies migrate in order to escape the pollens that proliferate in the damper, greener areas back of east-coast America. The next morning the woman awoke, sat up in her sleeping bag, stretched, and started to sneeze. She proceeded to sneeze her way through Arizona into Nevada, across California, on into Oregon and Washington, then most of the way home to New York; and to my knowledge she is still sneezing somewhere today. This woman was carrying around a potential sensitivity to a particular antigen for many years, perhaps most of her life. One day that potential became actual.

Yet here's the rub. While allergies may develop at any age in a person's lifetime, there is a greater tendency – a *far* greater tendency – for them to start up during childhood. Why? Partly because a child's immune system is more active and sensitive than an adult's. This means that not only are school-age children more likely than adults to acquire allergies, but so are infants, even the youngest. Indeed, the various digestive problems and skin rashes infants develop in the first months of life may be the result of allergic reactions to their diet. New parents should be aware that certain symptoms in newborn babies such as nasal stuffiness, chronic cough, and extreme irritability may ultimately be traced to allergic causes.

IT ALL STARTS IN THE IMMUNE SYSTEM

The main function of the immune system is to defend the body against invasion by bacteria, viruses, and assorted troublemaking foreign substances; also to eliminate any abnormal cells within the body that are potentially cancerous. During the course of our lifetime, millions and millions of these antigens enter our bodies; as you are reading this paragraph, numbers of them are entering yours and being processed by your immune system, pounced on and eliminated. People in whom this immune surveillance system is not working properly, such as those with AIDS, become ready targets of practically any unfriendly bacteria, often succumbing to germs which to a healthy immune mechanism would present nothing more challenging than a routine house-cleaning job.

The immune system is the body's principal defence force. Its various components are scattered throughout the body. Collectively, the thymus gland, spleen, tonsils, adenoids, lymph nodes (especially those in the intestinal tract), and bone marrow are the main parts of this 'system'. The cells that are the front-line fighters of this protective system are special white blood cells called lymphocytes.

Lymphocytes are produced in the bone marrow and then mature in either the thymus gland or the lymphoid tissue of the intestinal tract. These lymphocytes have special abilities and are able to protect you and me against bacteria, viruses, and cancerous cells.

What characterizes the sensitization process? When a child has become sensitized, it means that a specific type of white blood cell within his or her system, called a plasma cell, has been stimulated to produce a special protein known as an antibody. These antibodies circulate freely throughout the child's body; when they happen to meet certain foreign substances which have entered the body – that is, when they come in contact with allergens – an *allergic* reaction results. This response in turn takes place on the surface of another type of white blood cell called a mast cell. During the reaction the mast cells release a relatively large number of chemical compounds collectively called mediators; the best-known of these is histamine, the chemical culprit responsible for most of the sneezing, streaming eyes and sniffing that exasperate so many of us every year.

How many lymphocytes are there in your body right now? While precise counts are impossible to make, there are probably at any given time about a billion lymphocytes in the human organism capable of producing another million trillion antibodies. Indeed, in the time it has taken you to read this page your body has already produced millions of antibody molecules, each one unique, like snowflakes.

Each time your child is exposed to a new antigen – be it a food, virus or pollen grain – a group of these special antibodies is produced to confront this *specific* foreign substance and react with it. When substance A enters your body, your immune system produces antibodies specially engineered to deal with substance A; when substance B arrives, a new group of antibodies is created to deal exclusively with substance B, and so on. Our protective system – our immunological police force, if you will – is our main line of defence against all invaders from the outer world.

In a healthy child the immunological police force is on duty twenty-four hours a day, ever on the lookout for invaders. Usually the outcome between an antigen and its specific antibody is a foregone conclusion, with the antibody neatly overcoming the offending substance and routinely removing it. But in the case of an allergy something goes awry: the immune system becomes more of a problem than the foreign object it is attacking – usually nothing more than a harmless pollen or an innocuous food substance – and ends up provoking symptoms worse than anything these innocent substances might cause in a nonsensitized individual. Instead of blocking the development of symptoms, the immune system causes them. Antibodies are produced that do not protect the body. They actually have the opposite effect, serving as the triggers of allergic symptoms. An allergic reaction is, in brief, a protective mechanism gone haywire.

WHY CAN'T JOHNNY BREATHE?

Watch what happens during the course of a normal immune

response. Assume, for example, that Billy, aged four, has just started nursery school. In his second week in this 'public' environment he is exposed to virus A, causing him to develop an upper respiratory infection. Because Billy is in good health, his immune system easily deals with the virus and he recovers within four or five days.

Billy has now been exposed to virus A and his immunological lines of defence have produced antibodies against it. Next time virus A enters Billy's body, his immune system will 'remember' that it was once in contact with the bug and will produce large numbers of antibodies to block or blunt the virus from causing another respiratory infection.

Fine. Now, take the same child again. This time, though, Billy is experiencing an allergic reaction. See how his immune response misbehaves.

At first the same immunological sequence follows as with virus A. An allergen – in this case a pollen grain – lands on the mucous membrane inside Billy's nose. Blood cells called macrophages present in nearby nasal tissues take this grain, process it, and 'show' it to lymphocytes, which then produce antibodies to get rid of it.

The particular antibodies now produced, however, especially in a susceptible, genetically primed child like Billy, are of a special class. They are called *IgE immunoglobulins*.

Usually nonallergic children have very low levels of IgE immunoglobulin antibodies in their bloodstream and are not affected by them. Children reactive to a particular allergen, however, will begin producing IgE antibodies in great abundance whenever they come in contact with this allergen. As these antibodies proliferate they attach themselves to the surface of certain white blood cells, called basophil cells, which live in the bloodstream, and to mast cells, which are primarily located within the body tissues. Once this process occurs these mast and basophil cells are said to be 'sensitized', and henceforth when exposed to the specific allergen both will become the site of an allergic response.

Now mast cells and basophils are filled with many dense granules throughout their cellular substance, each granule enclosed by a membrane which insulates its chemical compounds from the rest of the cell. These chemical compounds are known as mediators.

Most mediators have chemical names unfamiliar to the layman. There is one which you're probably quite familiar with if there is allergy in your family. It is called histamine, and it is responsible for many of the common symptoms plaguing allergy sufferers. This troublesome chemical is released from the granules when the interaction just discussed takes place between IgE antibodies and the allergen. Once released, it seeps into surrounding local tissues and blood vessels, where it causes swelling and congestion, triggering the maddening itching sensations associated with skin allergies. In the lungs, histamine will narrow the breathing passages, sometimes throwing the victim into a full-fledged asthmatic spasm. In the nose it may cause nasal mucus glands to spew out a watery discharge; in the eyes it produces swollen lids and stinging tears; in the head it will stimulate headaches and sinus congestion; in the stomach, cramps and diarrhoea may occur. The more histamine there is in a particular area, the more acute the allergic reaction becomes. It's no fun.

These are the bare mechanics of allergy. In a mild reaction the symptoms can be controlled with nothing stronger than an over-the-counter antihistamine (note: *anti*histamine). In other situations allergic reactions take a more serious turn, especially when breathing is impaired or skin rashes get out of hand. At such times a doctor's help is decidedly in order.

CHAPTER TWO

Visiting the Doctor

IDENTIFYING YOUR CHILD'S SYMPTOMS

A runny nose, watery eyes, a sore throat, may all be due to hay fever. Or they may stem from a cold; the symptoms are almost identical. A breathing problem is the result of pollen sensitivity. Or is it a more serious disease? Or then again, perhaps it's just lingering bronchitis. The whole area of symptoms can get downright confusing, especially when many of these disparate symptoms appear simultaneously. How do you as a parent decide whether or not an allergy is behind it all?

Parents can make several valuable clinical observations when the question of allergic involvement arises. Short of a doctor's analysis, they are among the most efficient diagnostic resources a parent can know about.

Start by looking for *repeating patterns of symptoms* (listed opposite) *that tend to occur at regular intervals*, especially during specific months or seasons. Spring and autumn are the most likely times for such patterns to surface. They can, however, come at any time, cold or hot, rain or shine.

Then look for a pattern of symptoms that repeat under identical circumstances. For example, each time young Barbara eats a slice of bread, she starts to wheeze. This should cast suspicion on wheat. Every time Tom stretches out on his down-stuffed quilt, he sneezes. This may indicate an allergy to feathers.

Several years ago a young married couple and their five-year-old daughter moved from a small city in Iran to Boston. Within several months the child began to have regular sneezing bouts and to develop skin rashes, something she had never done before. The parents noted that the child's rash worsened after trips to a local playground. Following careful observation, the parents discovered that their daughter's reaction was caused by contact with dogs. As it happened, the child had grown up in a town without dogs of any kind. In the United States, her five-year-old heart became enchanted by the friendly creatures, so much so that she ran up and embraced every one that came near her on the playground. This frequent contact caused her to become sensitized to the animal's dander, and soon afterwards her symptoms appeared. This girl had the potential to react allergically to dogs, but the symptoms did not become apparent until she had repeated exposure to them.

Look for a set pattern of symptoms such as sneezing, nasal congestion or cough that becomes *chronic*. Be suspicious of a cold that drags on month after month; it probably isn't a cold at all. Or a cough that won't go away, or an annoying, itchy, persistent rash. Generally speaking, a viral or bacterial infection rarely lasts more than one or two weeks at a time, maximum; an allergy can go on for months or even years. If coldlike symptoms continue for five or six weeks, such lingering discomfort should put you on guard. More than likely you're looking at an allergic response.

What exactly are allergic symptoms? Though I will, of course, go into this question in some detail when examining the various specific allergic conditions in the sections that follow, a brief run-through here of the most common symptoms, taken organ by organ, will help you make your observations more quickly.

THE MOST COMMON ALLERGIC SYMPTOMS

The skin An allergic reaction involving the skin typically appears as a rash that is almost always very itchy. There is no consistent appearance for such an allergic rash. Anything from a red raised wheal, a typical hive, to the raw, oozing, reddened rash of acute eczema can result from an allergic response.

The eyes Symptoms include redness of the conjunctiva (the white portion of the eye), weeping and itching, swelling of the upper and lower lids, and the production of a gelatinous mucus secretion.

The nose Foremost, of course, is the runny nose. How to tell if it's from an allergy or a cold? One clue is that the nasal discharge caused by an allergy has a thin, clear, watery consistency, while the discharge from a cold or flu is thick, whitish, and heavy. A second observation is that even though children run about for weeks on end with a leaking nose, if the symptom is from an allergy the child will generally *not* develop an irritation of the upper lip and the nostrils, while children suffering from a viral or bacteria-caused nasal drip will.

Another important nasal symptom is sneezing. The child will tell you that there seems to be something blocking his nose. He can't smell very well or breathe through his nose. If a child sniffs constantly and wipes his nose with a passion, sometimes so frequently that the skin becomes raw, chances are he's allergic.

The mouth Look for complaints that the top (roof) of the mouth itches and futile attempts to use the tongue in order to get relief from this maddening symptom. There are also complaints of a sensation that something is constantly dripping down the back of the throat. This is called a postnasal drip.

The ears Allergic symptoms include a sensation of dripping within the ear, or itchiness, or of a feeling that the ears are clogged. A pre-speech child may tug on her earlobes, rub the side of her head, or frequently cock her head to one side. A child who can talk may tell you that she seems to hear things 'through water' – which is almost the case. At times the external portions of the ear may become reddened. Infants with hearing difficulties due to allergy will often show signs of language development problems. They may be late talkers, if they talk much at all, and you may notice that they have trouble relating easily with their peers.

The chest Watch for recurrent cough unassociated with other signs of a cold. There may be shortness of breath and an inability to take a deep breath. Also, a sensation of tightness in the chest accompanied by a whistling wheeze heard most often when the child is breathing out is the most typical symptom of asthma. The child may also complain of a pain in the chest, usually associated with prolonged coughing or when taking a deep breath. This pain is caused by stretching the muscles between the ribs and is common during an asthma attack.

The gastrointestinal tract The most frequent symptoms consist of nausea, vomiting and diarrhoea. A child who is having an asthma attack may complain of abdominal pain, which is caused by the diaphragm being forced downwards on to the stomach. When a young child has an asthma attack he may swallow large amounts of air, resulting in distension of and pain in the stomach.

Generalized allergic response An allergic reaction does not always occur in only one area. It may strike many parts of the body simultaneously in the form of a *generalized* response or, as it is known technically, anaphylaxis. Anaphylaxis is caused by a massive release of chemical mediators in many organ systems *all at the same time* with possible involvement of the lungs (wheezing, breathing difficulties), skin (generalized hives and swelling), intestinal tract (vomiting, diarrhoea) and the vascular system (drop in blood pressure with possible loss of consciousness). In other words, practically the entire body is affected. When a severe generalized reaction occurs, waste no time – *the outcome can be fatal if the condition is not given immediate medical attention.*

WHEN SHOULD YOU VISIT A DOCTOR?

When does an allergic problem become serious enough to warrant a trip to the doctor? This depends on two basic factors: the *frequency* of the child's symptoms and their *severity*.

Though it is difficult to make absolute recommendations, a good rule of thumb is this: if a child's symptoms can be controlled by using over-the-counter anti-allergic drugs such as antihistamines and decongestants, then no additional medical consultation may be necessary. If these drugs do not work, then a doctor should be consulted. If the symptoms are worsening, either in duration or in severity, stop medicating the child yourself and get immediate medical advice.

GENERAL PRACTITIONER OR ALLERGIST?

Sometimes, of course, parents suspect that their child's problem is an allergic one but do not know for certain. In this case a visit to the family doctor to discuss the situation is certainly appropriate. If he or she can relieve the child's symptoms with medication, which is often the case, then a trip to the specialist is unnecessary. Most allergy problems in this country are not treated by allergists; the treatment is quite well managed by the GP.

In some cases, however, the child's allergic problem will prove complicated or difficult. The GP may then feel that it is necessary to turn the case over to someone specially trained in this area of medicine. Enter the allergist.

An allergist is a doctor who has undergone a period of specialized training in the recognition, evaluation and treatment of clinical allergy and immunology problems. A referral is usually indicated when your child's symptoms are not responding to the treatment recommended by the family doctor, or the allergic symptoms persist and actually seem to be increasing in intensity.

In other words, if your child is experiencing continual or worsening symptoms, I feel it is appropriate to visit an allergist for a consultation. If there is an ongoing problem, I do not feel it is wise to wait on the chancy grounds that your child may 'outgrow' the condition. I have definite reservations about any doctor who assures parents that their child will outgrow his or her allergy. If there is no obvious improvement of your child's suspected problem, you should take it upon yourself at the very least to get a second medical opinion. While it is certainly true that many young children with significant allergy problems will lose their symptoms as they grow older, I certainly don't know how to predict who will be the lucky ones, and I have yet to meet the doctor who has the ability to see into the future!

REFERRAL TO AN ALLERGIST

Your family doctor may decide that the problem is too complicated for him or her to tackle without the help of a consultant, or you may feel that he or she has not made sufficient progress, and want a second opinion. There is no need to feel embarrassed about asking to be referred to a consultant. A good family doctor will not feel insulted by such a request; GPs know that they cannot be expert in all specialities and should be willing to seek specialist advice when they find themselves out of their depth.

A paediatrician (specialist in the illnesses of children) may be the first choice of consultant by your family doctor, especially if your child's illness involves factors other than allergy, but if allergic factors predominate your doctor may send you to an allergist. Since allergy is a relatively minor speciality there may not be an allergist at your local hospital, especially if it is a small one, and if this is so you may have to be sent to a larger centre. The services of an allergist are open to you under the NHS, or you may prefer to go privately. The actual treatment will be the same under both systems, but private medicine gives you more convenience of appointments, comfort in surroundings and possibly a more leisurely consultation. If you have private medical insurance you should be eligible for reimbursement of the consultation fees.

It is best to take the advice of your family doctor as to which specialist to go to, as he and the specialist have to work together and may well have built up a working relationship over the years. However, if you have been recommended to a particular specialist by a friend or relative, do not feel hesitant to put this idea forward and discuss it with your doctor, who should be prepared to take your wishes into consideration.

WHAT DOES AN ALLERGIST DO?

At the initial visit an allergist will require a highly detailed history of the child's present symptoms and medical past. This personal evaluation is the single most important diagnostic tool in the allergist's arsenal. All that is up-to-date and miraculous in modern laboratory technology is not worth the paper this page is printed on unless it comes coupled with a thorough description of your child's physical, social and psychological past. And you as parent are responsible for this description. The better organized this history is, the more detailed and complete, the more it will help your child.

After the child's detailed history is taken – more on this below – a complete physical examination is made, followed by medical tests when appropriate. These tests may run the gamut from a simple blood sample to sophisticated X-ray studies with many, many possibilities in between. We will look at some of the more common tests.

After all this input – the history, the physical examination, and the laboratory evaluation – has been weighed and considered, the doctor will make the final diagnosis of the child's condition and outline an appropriate programme of treatment. In some cases a limited course of medication to control symptoms is all that is required. In others, a variety of treatments will be called for including allergy injections, dietary manipulation, environmental control measures and special prescription medicines. The thoughtful allergist will design a treatment programme for your child that provides him with the maximum medical benefit and yet does not place an undue economic or logistical burden on the patient and family.

PREPARING FOR THE FIRST VISIT TO AN ALLERGIST

Bear in mind that a good allergist or a paediatrician will insist on including both parent(s) and child as integral parts of the doctor-parent-patient triangle. This relationship is the cornerstone of a successful partnership and will be crucial in guaranteeing the best possible results. Many chronic allergic conditions necessitate a long-term ongoing relationship between doctor and family. This relationship must be founded on the concept that while the doctor is the coach, everyone is an important part of the team. It must by no means be orchestrated by an aloof autocrat who sits behind a mahogany desk, writing mysterious prescriptions and issuing orders. If the doctor you're seeing never seems to have enough time for you, if he doesn't encourage your questions or if he answers the ones you manage to slip in with condescension or, worse, unintelligible 'doctorese', then you're probably involved with the wrong person. Consider looking elsewhere before a formal long-term commitment is made.

At the same time, parents must play their part. Those who

are not taking the time to formulate important questions before they visit their doctor are not doing their job. Those who allow the doctor to do all the talking and all the thinking, who fail to keep a watchful eye on their child's condition at home and who do not consider themselves as a fundamental part of the healing unit are missing an important opportunity to help everyone involved. What is most important in the doctor-patient-parent partnership is the free flow of ideas, the sharing of observations, and a mutual commitment to the patient. If one partner remains uninvolved, the whole therapeutic programme automatically fails.

I strongly advise that at your first visit to an allergist you come prepared to participate in all decisions and to share the important facts of your child's past medical history. I suggest that you sit down several days before the first visit, either by yourself or, better, with your spouse, and write down significant facts related to your child's allergic past. The more prepared you are to answer the doctor's questions at the first visit, the more immediate feedback he will be able to give you. Here is a checklist of the possible questions the doctor may ask concerning your child's personal allergic history, to which you should have answers ready.

A CHECKLIST OF YOUR CHILD'S HISTORY

What was the date of the child's first attack?

What were the specific circumstances involved at the time of this attack? Did the child eat something new, breathe something unusual, rub something exotic on his skin? Was he bitten or stung? If so, by what?

Where was the child when the first attack occurred? In the city? The country? At home? In the playground? At the cinema? At the house of a friend? In school?

During what time of year were the symptoms noticed?

What medical treatment, if any, was provided?

What was the apparent outcome of the treatment?

How long did this first bout of allergy last?

The question of how the symptoms have evolved since their initial onset will be of key importance in this history:

How often do the symptoms now occur?

Do the symptoms tend to appear when the child is in one specific geographic location – in rural areas, in urban areas, at home, by the sea, etc.? Does the condition improve when the child travels from one geographic area to another – i.e., from the seaside to the city, from hilly country to low-lying areas, etc.?

How severe is the attack when it occurs? In what physical and psychological ways does the child react?

Describe all the symptoms of the suspected allergic response, even those that seem insignificant or secondary. In what part of the body are they predominantly located?

Is the child's condition stable at present? Does it seem to be getting worse? Is it improving?

Are there any differences in symptoms during the day and during the night? At what time of day are the symptoms most intense? Is there a specific seasonal pattern to the problem: is it worse during one particular time of year, better during another?

Then the question of diet:

What in general does the child eat? How closely can you describe your child's average daily menu?

Do you know of any particular foods that seem to cause allergic symptoms? Which foods are generally disliked? Which ones are most enjoyed and most frequently eaten?

If the child is thought to be allergic to certain foods, how long does it take for the reaction to set in? Which organs are affected? In what way?

What drugs were taken during pregnancy? Was the child breastfed? If not, what formula was used?

Also important is information regarding previous medical consultations and the child's general medical history:

What medical treatments have been given in the past for allergic symptoms? For how long were they taken? Give the specific names of the medicines prescribed, and the doses. (Descriptions such as 'a blue pill' or 'a clear liquid' are practically worthless. Provide the actual *names* of the medicines, either from the pharmacist who supplied them or the doctor who prescribed them; both parties should have this information on record.)

Have there been any problems related to the medications?

Have any prior laboratory tests been made? What were the results? If possible the results from any previous test should be brought to the consultation at the time of the first visit. Copies or summaries of consultations can be obtained by contacting the original doctor and requesting that he or she forward the records to the allergist.

Be prepared to discuss the child's family history:

What are the parent's occupations? Has the child any brothers and sisters? Do any of them have a history of allergy?

Is there a record of allergy in the family? (This means not only the father and mother but grandparents, brothers and sisters, even uncles, aunts and cousins.) How badly do any of these family members suffer from this ailment?

Is there any unusual medical history in the family? Are there other chronic conditions the doctor should be informed of?

Have there been unusual family problems that have gone undiagnosed?

Has the child ever been hospitalized? If so, what for?

What kind of immunizations have been given in the past?

What was the mother's pregnancy with the child like? Were there any noteworthy incidents or problems, especially feeding problems, during the first few months of life?

You should also be prepared to describe the immediate environment that presently surrounds your child. This applies especially to your home and all the many things in it:

How old is your house?

What kind of heating system do you have? If your heating system is forced air, how often do you change the filters? Do you use humidifiers? Do you have air conditioning?

Is your basement dry? Damp? Does your child frequent this area very often?

What are your pillows made of? Your carpets? Your blankets? Does anyone in your home work with strong chemicals such as the paints, glues or photographic substances used by hobbyists? Do you live near any industrial plants?

Is your child ever exposed to unusual substances at a childminder's home or play group?

What about the child's toys? Are they stuffed or made of unusual materials? What objects does the child sleep with at night? Which toys are played with most during the day?

Do you have a pet in the house? What type? These include the less conspicuous varieties such as birds and hamsters as well as cats and dogs. How much contact does the child have with the animal? How long have you owned it? Have you ever noted any strange reactions on the child's part after the child and the pet have been together for a period of time?

How dry, dust-free and chemical-free is the child's room, especially the area where she sleeps? Is there a carpet on the floor? What type of material is the carpet made of? How recently has the room been painted? What type of paint was used?

Parents should come to their first visit with questions of their own. Draw up a list before you arrive. Consider all the many questions you've asked yourself through the years concerning your child's condition; jot them down. Some of these questions may be unanswerable on the first visit, and some may never be answerable. But you should ask anything you like, and usually there will be answers.

Briefly, you can hope for all of the following from an allergist's evaluation:

A decision regarding the allergic or nonallergic cause of your child's symptoms.

A specific recommendation or plan of treatment for the child's condition. In general, allergies cannot be cured. But with the forms of treatment available today, most can be very well controlled.

Perhaps most important, a sympathetic ear and a dependable source of information that can provide answers from the knowledge of direct experience.

On the other hand, allergists cannot predict the future. Neither at the first meeting nor at any other time can an allergist say with certainty whether a child will get better, get worse or stay the same. He cannot predict whether your child will respond positively to a specific form of treatment or outgrow his symptoms.

What the allergist *can* promise you is that he will provide you with informed, conscientious service and that the most up-to-date and effective methods of modern medicine will be made available to your child. In most cases the combination of these two powerful tools will lead to a successful outcome. In most cases a child can and will be helped.

CHAPTER THREE

Evaluating the Allergic Child

PERSONAL HISTORY AND PHYSICAL EXAMINATION

Personal history, physical examination, laboratory tests: of the three the personal history is usually the most important. It should be detailed and very specific. Some doctors ask parents for an oral history, while others provide a form for the family to fill in at the time of the initial examination or before the first consultation. If you are asked to fill in one of these forms, be as thorough as possible. A study of the personal history checklist in the preceding chapter will help you.

After the history has been obtained, the doctor will then perform a physical examination of your child. In preparation for this experience, explain to the young person that this part of the visit does not hurt at all. Ever. That it will be more or less like any other examination at any other doctor's surgery and nothing drastic or bizarre will take place. Height and weight will be checked; the eyes, nose, mouth, and ears will be looked at; the doctor will listen to the heartbeat, examine the skin, take blood pressure, and so on. For the youngest patients it is good psychology to let them touch the medical instruments like the stethoscope or otoscope before the examination begins, to demonstrate their harmlessness. Usually the examination will last no longer than fifteen minutes.

ALLERGY TESTS AND HOW THEY WORK

After the history and physical examination are completed, tests will usually be ordered appropriate to the specific allergic problem. There are, of course, a goodly number of these, the most important of which we will discuss now, close up, from the standpoint of what you should know concerning how these tests work, why they are ordered, what they determine, the ways in which they are administered to the child, the dangers or pain involved, and any other significant facts.

Most allergists' tests are quickly administered and relatively pain-free. Still, it is well within your rights as concerned parent, should you wish it, to request a list of the tests that your child will undergo and to familiarize yourself with it. You can then check this list against the description of allergy tests given below to understand better how they work, and why a certain procedure has been ordered for your child.

A CHECKLIST OF ALLERGY TESTS

BLOOD TESTS

Full blood count

PURPOSE Frequently a full blood count or FBC will be done to check the overall condition of the blood. A low haemoglobin level indicates that some form of anaemia is present. If the white blood cell count is elevated, there may be an infection. This test helps the doctor determine whether the child's symptoms stem from a bacterial/viral infection or from an allergic sensitivity.

FREQUENCY Standard. It is usually done on the first visit and may be repeated at infrequent intervals.

HOW ADMINISTERED An FBC can be done in two ways: either by pricking the child's finger and taking a smear, or by removing blood directly via a needle (a process called *venipuncture*). Both are usually done by a technician in a laboratory.

PAIN Both are associated with mild discomfort, though neither is very painful. The venipuncture is probably more menacing, simply because it involves a hypodermic needle.

RESULTS AVAILABLE In one or two days at most.

Quantitative immunoglobulins determination test

PURPOSE Here the doctor is looking for three different immuno-globulin proteins: IgG, IgA and IgM (the Ig stands for immu-noglobulin). These antibody proteins are normally produced by all of us and are a regular part of the body's immune system. Some children with abnormally low levels of these proteins, specifically IgG, have a tendency to develop severe bacterial infections. Your doctor may suspect that a patient's pattern of repeated infections is associated with such an abnormality, and the gammaglobulin level will give him important information about this aspect of the body's defence mechanism. The test will provide evidence of a deficiency of the immune system.

FREQUENCY Not on a regular basis; generally performed when there is a problem with repeated infections. Usually the test will be performed only once if the results are normal.

HOW ADMINISTERED By a venipuncture or finger stick. If a child requires both the FBC and a quantitative immunoglobulins test, blood is drawn only once; both tests will then be made from the single sample.

PAIN Usually mild and momentary when performed by a skilled technician or doctor.

RESULTS AVAILABLE In several days to a week.

Serum IgE level determination

PURPOSE Done quite frequently today, an IgE level determination, like the quantitative immunoglobulins determination test, searches for a specific immunoglublin protein in the blood – in this case the IgE protein. IgE was first discovered in 1967 and has since been found to be a specific marker for the presence of allergic disease. While an elevation of the IgE in the blood does not invariably accompany allergic problems, approximately 60 to 70 per cent of people who have allergic symptoms will also have an increased IgE level, and that's a pretty fair percentage. Examining a blood sample from this perspective, a doctor can thus come to a more definitive conclusion about symptoms which look suspiciously like allergy – runny nose, sneezing, etc. – but which can also stem from non-allergic causes.

FREQUENCY A standard allergy test.

HOW ADMINISTERED Through venipuncture.

PAIN Momentary discomfort.

RESULTS AVAILABLE In several days.

COMMENTS The IgE will not tell the doctor specifically *what* the person is allergic to, only that with an elevated IgE level there is a very good chance the person *is* allergic. Almost all people suffering from atopic dermatitis will have a high IgE level.

X-RAYS

Conventional X-ray study

VARIETIES The doctor may request a number of X-ray studies. Here are the four most common ones:

Chest X-ray taken from the back and the side, called PA and lateral views. The child will be asked to take a deep breath so that the lungs are fully expanded. Some time before the X-ray is scheduled it is a good idea for parents to make the child practise taking a deep breath, holding it as the parents count to three, and then exhaling. Any child with a history of recurring or persistent chest symptoms including chronic cough, wheeze, shortness of breath, and persistent tightness of chest is a candidate for a chest X-ray.

Sinus X-rays. May be ordered when there are recurring episodes of dizziness and pain located in the forehead and under the eyes, or for symptoms of chronic foul-smelling nasal discharge. In general, sinus X-rays will not be ordered for children under five, as these areas are not sufficiently developed in younger children. The radiologist will examine the X-rays for the presence of fluid within the sinuses, indicating improper drainage and the probability of infection; blockage of the sinus passages resulting from recurring infection; cysts or polyps growing in the sinus areas; thickening of the membranes lining the sinuses (a sign of either chronic infection or allergic stimulation).

Side or lateral X-ray view of the neck. May be done as a check for chronically enlarged adenoids. Not ordered very often.

Upper or lower intestinal tract X-rays. Used to evaluate the presence of chronic gastrointestinal complaints such as vomiting, nausea, diarrhoea which might possibly have an allergic cause, i.e., from a food allergy. A barium containing contrast material is swallowed and films are then taken.

PURPOSE To search for the cause of specific stomach or intestinal complaints.

HOW ADMINISTERED By conventional X-ray equipment.

FREQUENCY With chronic chest complaints an X-ray is frequently ordered. Sinus films are taken in older children and adolescents with persistent headaches. Gastrointestinal films are done infrequently, generally only with chronic or severe stomach or intestinal complaints.

PAIN None.

COMMENTS Though the safety of X-ray technology has been immensely improved through the years, it is still sound policy to ask the doctor what information she hopes to obtain from this test. Be very sceptical if the doctor's answer is too general or too vague. Any patient who enters the consulting room with mild chest symptoms and some nasal symptoms should not be sent for X-rays immediately. If an X-ray study has been done recently, it may be unnecessary to repeat it.

Barium swallow

PURPOSE To find any unusual anatomical relationship existing between the feeding pathway (the oesophagus) and the air passageway (the trachea); to find an improperly functioning junction at the point where the oesophagus meets the stomach; to find an abnormal connection between the oesophagus and the trachea, the result being the formation of an anatomical abnormality known as a tracheo-oesophageal (T-E) fistula; if such a connection has formed, food may be backing up into the lungs, causing symptoms which cannot be readily distinguished from those of asthma. Gastro-oesophageal reflux, another condition that can cause asthma symptoms, can be diagnosed with a barium swallow.

HOW ADMINISTERED The child is asked to swallow a chalky barium mixture. The mixture is then X-rayed as it moves down the oesophagus to the stomach; this is like a standard X-ray except that many more exposures are made at a single session and the test may last for up to thirty minutes.

FREQUENCY This test is ordered only when the doctor is suspicious that a fistula exists or the gastro-oesophageal junction is not functioning properly.

PAIN No pain of any kind. The young child may, however, becomes restless or uncomfortable during the picture-taking session. The chocolate-flavoured barium mixture is usually quite palatable to the child.

Magnification X-rays of upper airways

PURPOSE To examine with magnification the trachea and main branches of the bronchial tubes. The test is used to get an enlarged view of the anatomy of the major breathing passage-ways. This procedure can detect a variety of congenital structural abnormalities such as vascular rings, which can compress the oesophagus and trachea.

FREQUENCY Uncommon. Usually this test is called for only when there is suspicion that a foreign object has been swallowed – coins, food, a blade of grass – and that this object has become lodged in the airways, producing asthma-like symptoms.

PAIN None.

IN VITRO TESTS

The term *in vitro* literally means 'in a glass' or 'in a test tube' –

figuratively, it describes a procedure that takes place in an environment *outside* the body. In vitro tests are therefore carried out in a laboratory rather than being performed directly on the patient.

RAST test (radioallergosorbent test)

PURPOSE An in vitro technique for measuring the circulating level of a specific IgE antibody (e.g. anti-mould IgE antibody) in the bloodstream. This test determines the level of potential sensitivity to a variety of specific allergens, including pollens, animals, moulds, foods, and inhalants.

HOW ADMINISTERED By venipuncture. The blood sample is divided into many small test tubes, each containing a different antigen, e.g. pollen, mould, dog dander, dust, wool, milk, etc. These specimens are then analysed in a machine designed to detect either colour changes in the tested substance or the degree of radioactivity in each tube. The procedure is performed using a system that detects changes in the colour of a particular test sample or by means of radioactively tagged allergens.

PAIN Mild momentary discomfort.

HOW COMMON A frequently performed test.

COMMENTS The appeal of RAST testing is that many tests can be performed from one blood specimen; a doctor can identify a wide spectrum of possible allergic sensitivities from analysis of a single laboratory sample, making it unnecessary for the child to return for further tests. The disadvantages of RAST testing are that the method is less sensitive than direct skin testing (see below) and a good deal more expensive.

IN VIVO OR DIRECT SKIN TESTS

Skin tests performed directly on the patient are known as *in vivo* tests, i.e. tests carried out on a person rather than in the lab.

Epicutaneous testing (skin tests)

PURPOSE To determine allergic sensitivities to specific allergens.

HOW ADMINISTERED By scratch, and prick technique.

The *scratch test* is done by making a row of superficial (and bloodless) scratches on the skin with a needle. A drop of a specific antigen extract – dog extract, shellfish extract, etc. – is placed directly on one of the scratches and absorbed. A different antigen is then placed on the second scratch, another on the third, and so on. Each test site is numbered or otherwise labelled so that the antigen can be identified. Ten of these scratches may be made at one time on the forearm, or in some cases along the upper part of the back, usually in vertical rows. If the child has been sensitized to any of the specific allergens, a red, swollen hivelike bump will soon appear at that specific test site. The degree of reaction is then graded on a one-to-four scale: the larger, redder and more dramatic the bump, the greater the sensitivity. Twenty, or at most, thirty scratch tests may be done at a single testing session.

In the prick technique, a drop of antigen is placed on the forearm. The test site is then pricked with a needle, allowing the antigen to make contact with the tissue mast cells. A positive response consists of localized itching, swelling and redness on the test site. The patient who demonstrates such a reaction has been sensitized to the specific test substance placed on that spot. Ten to thirty prick tests can be done during a consultation. The usual test site is the forearm. Prick testing is a somewhat more sensitive method than scratch testing and is probably the best of all in vivo methods for food testing.

These tests are administered in the allergist's consulting room. If reactions occur, they usually take place within ten to twenty minutes after the tests have been performed.

HOW COMMON A standard allergist's test. Both the scratch and the prick tests are first-line diagnostic allergy procedures, and they are effective techniques. When direct food testing is done, the prick test is the current method of choice.

PAIN The pain is no greater – and lasts no longer – than any other kind of scratch or pinprick. Most children take the momentary discomfort easily in their stride. In the hands of a competent, concerned doctor, anxiety and pain response are minimal.

POTENTIAL DANGERS Although there are rarely problems related to this type of testing, the child is being tested for substances to which she may be allergic. This means that in addition to the local response on the arm – which feels and looks no worse than a large mosquito bite – the test material on rare occasions may trigger a more generalized allergic reaction. When this occurs, symptoms can take many forms: hives, general itching, sneezing, weeping eyes, even asthma. Such a reaction is extremely rare and responds dramatically to treatment given in the allergist's consulting room.

COMMENTS The direct or in vivo skin test is one of the most sensitive and specific ways we have for detecting allergic sensitivities. A positive test indicates *only* that the patient has been *sensitized* to the test substance and therefore has the potential to develop allergic symptoms on re-exposure to that allergen. Understand that this is *not* incontrovertible proof of a clinical allergic sensitivity. To come to this conclusion the doctor must evaluate the entire history, physical condition and testing records of the child.

Intracutaneous or intradermal testing (literally, 'within the layers of skin')

PURPOSE To determine specific allergic sensitivities to particular allergens.

HOW ADMINISTERED An antigen is injected into the superficial layers of the skin. Injections are applied approximately an inch apart in rows on the forearm or occasionally the upper back. If a reaction takes place, it will occur ten to twenty minutes after the injection.

HOW COMMON A standard allergy testing procedure. Once this test has been performed, it is usually unnecessary to repeat it. Only if there is a *significant* change in the child's symptoms should he be called in for further testing. I have never understood why some patients have been tested on a yearly basis when there has been no worsening of their symptoms or obvious change in the clinical course. I can think of no scientific reason to justify the constant retesting of patients who are progressing satisfactorily.

PAIN Mild momentary discomfort. The pain associated with intradermal testing in the hands of a well-trained individual working with a co-operative patient usually causes minimal discomfort.

POTENTIAL DANGERS In order to minimize the possibility of either a large local reaction or a more generalized response, the testing is started with highly diluted allergen mixtures. None the less, the same small chance of a general allergic reaction that exists for epicutaneous testing (described above) is also present here.

COMMENTS The intracutaneous technique is the most sensitive of all skin tests, *except* in the case of food allergies, where false responses to tested materials are common. If skin testing for foods is to be done at all, the best method to employ is the prick technique.

Patch testing

PURPOSE Used to evaluate substances suspected of causing allergic-type skin problems. It is particularly effective in identifying the metal and chemical allergies which cause contact dermatitis.

HOW ADMINISTERED A piece of soft cloth or paper is impregnated with the suspected allergen. The patch is then applied directly to the skin of the patient's forearm or back and covered with an adhesive bandage-type dressing. The test substance is left on for forty-eight hours and then removed. A positive response consists of itching with redness and blistering of the skin at the test site.

FREQUENCY Patch testing is sometimes done by the allergist; however, more commonly it is performed in a dermatologist's consulting room. In general, an allergist may refer patients suffering from any unusual skin conditions to a dermatologist.

PAIN Rarely. The usual response consists of localized itching and possible blister formation at the test site.

Oral challenge food testing

PURPOSE To confirm a suspected allergic sensitivity to a particular food substance.

HOW ADMINISTERED Allergists do not yet have any totally accurate, easily performed testing methods for food allergies. The best system that exists is direct food challenge testing. This form of dietary manipulation calls for the removal of specific suspected foods or food groups from the child's diet: milk or oranges, for example. The patient is then observed to see if the allergic symptoms disappear. If symptoms do decrease, the patient is given the specific food again. If the symptoms reappear, this is good evidence of an allergic reaction. If the test is done twice with the same results, it is proof positive. In this case the expression 'the proof of the pudding is in the eating' is an especially appropriate motto.

PAIN If the test is positive, the patient can experience a variety of allergic symptoms.

HOW COMMON A standard test.

POTENTIAL DANGERS If the original reaction to the suspected food was very severe, with breathing problems, severe vomiting or diarrhoea, then it is potentially quite dangerous to carry out a direct food challenge test. If it is absolutely essential to do this test, it must be carried out under direct medical supervision, preferably in a hospital. In this situation a challenge procedure is definitely *not* a medical do-it-yourself project.

FREQUENTLY PERFORMED TESTS

Pulmonary function study

PURPOSE To judge how well the lungs are performing. Generally used by an allergist when dealing with asthmatic patients.

HOW ADMINISTERED The child is asked to breathe into a mechanical device of some kind; there are many varieties. Like blood pressure readings, 'normal' lung function values fall within a range which varies with a person's age, height, race and sex.

A child who suffers from asthma will probably have some abnormal lung function values, even if there have been no recent symptoms.

PAIN No pain.

HOW COMMON Commonly performed with asthmatic children. The test may be done repeatedly, throughout the child's course of treatment. It is now possible to get cheap plastic peak flow meters, one of the most common instruments used to measure pulmonary function, and there is a growing tendency to provide the patient with one. A peak flow meter can determine the need to vary the dose of medicaments for asthma.

COMMENTS A doctor may listen to a child's lungs through a stethoscope and find the patient's chest totally clear. This does not, however, indicate how well the child's lungs are actually functioning; a patient can have a serious asthma and between attacks have totally clear-sounding lungs.

Sweat test for cystic fibrosis

PURPOSE Cystic fibrosis, or CF, is a genetically transmitted disease in which there is an abnormality in such glandular organs as the pancreas, salivary glands, sweat glands and mucus glands of the intestinal and respiratory systems. The symptoms, which include a cough, production of very thick mucus secretions and occasional wheezing, can under certain circumstances mimic those seen in asthma. For this reason the presence of cystic fibrosis must first of all be ruled out in young children before proceeding to make a diagnosis of asthma.

HOW ADMINISTERED Children who are suffering from CF have exceedingly high levels of sodium chloride in their sweat. This imbalance can be detected by placing a piece of gauze on the child's arm and stimulating the sweat glands with a very low-grade electrical current. The wrapping is left on the arm for about an hour and then removed. The sweat content is analysed for the amount of sodium chloride it has produced.

HOW COMMON This test is necessary only if a child has chronic respiratory symptoms similar to those found in cystic fibrosis.

PAIN None.

AFTER THE TESTS ARE COMPLETED

Once the appropriate tests have been completed, the findings are used in conjunction with the child's history and examination records to reach a final diagnosis, and then to formulate a plan of treatment. This treatment may involve one or all of three main therapeutic approaches. These are: environmental control; pharmacotherapy, the use of a wide range of medicines to control the child's allergic symptoms; immunotherapy, or allergy injection treatment to build up the child's resistance and immunity to specific allergen(s).

We will go into all three forms of allergy treatment in the next chapter. Remember: the presence of a positive reaction to any allergen during a test does not *necessarily* mean that a child is actually allergic to this substance. It does mean that the child has at some point in his life been exposed to this particular allergen, and sensitization to this substance has occurred. Once the child has been sensitized, production of specific anti-dog IgE antibodies – or whatever – provides him with the capability to develop allergic symptoms to these specific substances. Such a response can take place today, tomorrow, in ten years, or never. One simply never knows. Yet how common it is for a young patient to walk out of my consulting room announcing: 'I'm allergic to trees, grass, and feathers', when all that has really been established is that she has tested positively to these substances. Only after a doctor has evaluated *all* the clinical evidence can the child, the parents, and the doctor be sure that an allergy is really present.

CHAPTER FOUR

How an Allergist Treats Your Allergic Child

ENVIRONMENTAL CONTROL

Whenever possible, the best way to stop allergic symptoms is to avoid the source of the problem. This approach is called environmental control. For example, if it has been determined that your child is allergic to dust or the pet dog, then elimination or avoidance of these allergens will be a big help in controlling symptoms. This sounds simple and pat, and it is. Yet it's amazing how many parents overlook environmental control, even when a few easy changes might remedy a lifetime of allergic misery. The fact is that many allergic children can significantly decrease their symptoms merely by having suspected allergens removed from their living area; or, in certain cases, by removing themselves from the problem area. Whenever it can be practised, preventive medicine is the best medicine.

For example, Richie, a thirteen-year-old boy, was recently brought to my consulting room because for the first time in his life he was experiencing severe allergic symptoms: sneezing, streaming eyes and a maddening itch in the back of his throat. These symptoms had come on suddenly and with surprising violence a month and a half before his visit, and they were now continuing day after day without let-up.

In the course of taking the boy's history I soon determined that one aspect of his life had changed: he had been given a long-haired collie about a month before his symptoms started. I did a skin test and found that the boy had a strong positive response to dog dander. I explained the situation to his family, and they all agreed to part with the dog on a trial basis. Within two weeks after the animal had left the home Richie's symptoms disappeared entirely.

Allergic symptoms do not always vanish with such ease, of course, and in many cases it is impossible to move away entirely from the source of an allergen. What cannot be avoided, however, can usually – I say *usually* – be manipulated, and this is the key to the practice of environmental control.

Dust, for example, is ubiquitous and a nemesis for millions of allergy-prone children. Contrary to popular notion, it is not composed of dirt or soil but a combination of the breakdown products of organic materials: animal dander, wool and linen fibres, feathers and plant residues. The dust in my house will be different from the dust in yours depending on how often you clean, whether you keep a pet, whether you raise plants, and so on.

One of the inhabitants of dust is an organism known as the dust mite, a quasi-microscopic insect that abides quite happily in the residences of rich and poor alike – it is no respecter of fine living. We all have an ample collection of these mites in our households, generally in the bedroom and specifically in our pillows, blankets and mattresses (the mites feed upon the tiny flakes of skin that fall from our bodies while we sleep). Disconcerting? Perhaps. But every home has its share of dust mites, and if kept policed they do no harm, except of course to those with dust allergies. For such people environmental control is imperative.

How can environmental control be carried out? In several ways.

ELECTRONIC AIR-CONTROLLED DEVICES

Various electronic devices may be used to make physical changes in the nature of the air. These are of relevance in countries that experience extremes of climatic conditions.

Air conditioners

These are used in countries which experience long torrid summers. They can be very useful in the homes of allergy sufferers, especially those sensitive to air-borne allergens such as dust, mould spores and pollens. Not only do they partially filter out particles of dust and pollen, they cool the air and lower its humidity. They need to be kept scrupulously clean and the filters need to be changed frequently or they may pump contaminated air back into the room.

While air conditioners are helpful, they tend to filter out only larger particulate matter, such as mould spores and some pollens. Some of the more efficient machines have the capacity to remove airborne allergens in the 10- to 15-micron range. To give you some idea of the relative size of a micron, there are 25 millimetres in an inch and one micron is equal to 1/1000 of a millimetre. It's not very large! Special air filtering devices are required to remove airborne particles smaller than 5 microns (cigarette smoke, bacteria and metallic fumes). If you want complete protection from such irritants, you'll need an electronic air cleaner to supplement your air conditioner.

Humidifiers and dehumidifiers

Many heating systems dry the air, robbing it of essential water vapour. Too much of this artificial dryness will eventually cause the protective mucus barrier in the nose and throat to crack, making the inhabitants of the household vulnerable to viral and bacterial infections. Schoolchildren who complain of sore throats during those months when the heating system is working are not necessarily malingering; they may simply be having difficulty differentiating between what is infected and what is irritated. The simplest and cheapest way of overcoming this condition is to stand relatively wide, shallow pans of water close to the heating units. However, special humidifying machines can be obtained. These put water vapour back into over-dry air and can be run regularly when the heating system is on. Look for a machine equipped with a *humidistat* which turns itself on and off automatically. The newest and most efficient room humidifier is the ultrasonic. The aerosol mist produced by this unit is so fine that it stays suspended in the air for long periods of time. Consequently the room does not become cold and damp, a condition that occurs quite often with other types of room humidifier. The ultrasonic units operate completely silently. This feature can be quite important for the child who has a problem falling asleep.

Between 35 and 45 per cent relative humidity is an ideal environment for human beings. Anything much above this and the atmosphere becomes predisposed to mould growth, especially undesirable in the home of any allergic child.

High humidity may also aggravate asthma symptoms; this is why some asthmatics are more uncomfortable during hot, humid weather. However, this type of condition seldom lasts long enough to make purchase of a dehumidifier necessary.

Vaporizers

Many householders use simple vaporizers, the most common type being the coal tar vaporizer. These are mainly used for the relief of nasal catarrh in small children and consist of a small night-light-type candle which heats up coal tar liquid and turns it into vapour.

The smell of coal tar vapour is characteristic and can be recognized on entering the house, as the clean tarry smell spreads everywhere. Not often seen now, but very effective in its day, was the old steam kettle which consisted of a simple kettle but with a long spout, the end of which was spread out into a fan shape. Its main use was for treating a child with croup, but nowadays it is easier to take the child into a heated steamed-up bathroom and this works well. Generally speaking, neither of these has much place in the home of an allergic child.

MANIPULATION OF THE EXTERNAL ENVIRONMENT

You can make many modifications in your child's surroundings, many of them simple and most of them surprisingly effective. In certain cases a few modifications may be *all* that is necessary to control allergic symptoms.

Make a household room check By carefully going through each room in your house or flat you can remedy many conditions which can aggravate or trigger allergy symptoms. The living room, for instance, usually has more furniture in it than any other room. Keep all tables, chairs, bookcases, blinds, curtains, couches and bric-a-brac dust free, and vacuum the rugs at least twice a week.

Watch out for wool-covered and overstuffed furniture, especially old furniture; both may be potential allergy hazards. You may wish to encase such furniture in protective coverings. In dens and offices, books are legendary collectors of dust if not gone over frequently with a rag or vacuum cleaner. Flocked wallpaper is also a potential allergic hazard because it attracts dust. Cooking odours from the kitchen may cause allergic symptoms; a good exhaust fan over the stove can remedy this problem. Bathroom tiles should be kept scrubbed and disinfected to eliminate mould, especially those located around the basin, bath and other damp spots. There are a number of effective sprays on the market that will kill moulds before they become a problem. Your local supermarket or hardware store will be able to supply you with the names of these products. Basement areas may hold pockets of dampness that contribute to mould growth, which a dehumidifer will eliminate. Clothes dryers should be adequately vented to prevent dust and lint from recirculating through the house. Each house is different, of course, and has different logistic problems. Check each room, and make appropriate modifications when needed.

Choose rugs and furnishings wisely If you're going to use carpeting in a child's room, make sure it is a low-pile, nonwool, synthetic variety. The padding beneath the rug should be made of foam rather than a hair-type material. Furniture is less likely to cause allergic symptoms if it is stuffed with foam rubber rather than kapok or feathers. Replace heavy curtains with washable ones. Avoid animal materials such as mohair, wool or horsehair.

Dustproof the child's bedroom Approximately half of a young child's day is spent in her bedroom, so the necessity for dustproofing an allergic child's bedroom is self-evident. Get rid of all pillows and mattresses stuffed with kapok or down and replace them with foam- or polyester-stuffed varieties. Upholstered box springs should be avoided; they attract dust. The ideal sleeping arrangement for an allergic child is a platform-style bed or a bed with metal springs with all pillows and box springs enclosed in dustproof casings. Special dustproof mattress covers are helpful too, but shun headboards covered with fabric or upholstery. The child's blankets should be made of polyester or cotton. Be careful of the woollen varieties – even if they do not promote allergies directly, they can be great dust catchers. Keep the door of the child's room closed when not occupied and try to vacuum the room at least every other day. Closed bookcases and cupboard doors that seal shut are helpful, as are washable curtains. Do not store toys or bric-a-brac under the bed or in any enclosed spot where dust accumulates and remove damp clothes from the room, as well as mothballs, plants, perfumes, insect sprays, and hobby chemicals such as glue and paint. Dust mites, incidentally, cannot survive extremely low temperatures: airing a child's mattress and bed coverings on a sunny winter day will have an antiseptic as well as a freshening effect. Vacuuming the mattress once a week will help reduce the dust mite population.

Maintain adequate temperature control Avoid extremes of heat and cold. In the winter the indoor temperature should be maintained between 20 and 22 degrees Centigrade (68 and 72 degrees Fahrenheit). In the summer, keeping the windows shut and the blinds drawn in really hot weather will stop the indoor temperature rising too high.

Clean your house often and with a special eye to reducing dust Clean all rooms thoroughly, especially those where the child spends much time. Always use the vacuum cleaner or a damp mop; avoid feather dusters or brooms. Disinfectants are all right for scrubbing, but first be sure the child is not allergic to them. Keep the child's room as uncluttered and airy as possible, and furnish it with substances posing no allergic danger: wood furniture; curtains of synthetic materials; plastic toys and furnishings; linoleum, wood, vinyl or tile floors; Formica desks and shelves; washable enamel paint on the walls, etc. Likewise, shun materials such as rattan, cane, velour, fur, wicker, mohair, wool, and so on, and be wary of stuffed animals. When vacuuming, don't forget to concentrate on the dust-catching areas such as beneath the bed and across the Venetian blinds. On major cleaning days it is wise for the child to leave the house for several hours because heavy cleaning raises the dust level temporarily.

Pets require special handling and consideration Children with sensitivities to animals are obviously best off when the animals are removed from the house. For a variety of reasons, however, most of them psychological, the child and the animal may be inseparable. In this case you must minimize contact. Vacuum the house frequently to remove animal hairs and shedding residues. The child's bedroom should be *absolutely, totally and always off-limits to the dog or cat*; and under *no* circumstances should the pet be allowed to sleep with the child or even climb up on his bed. The child must have an *absolutely animal-free sanctuary* in some section of the house for days when symptoms become intense, and if possible the animal should be housed outside much of the time.

Children are not allergic to animal hair or even to animal fur. What they are allergic to is the dander, the dead skin cells that constantly flake off the creature's body as the animal moves about. All animals produce dander, especially during the shedding season. This means, despite the claims of some animal breeders, that there is no such thing as a nonallergenic dog or cat. To make matters worse, many children are allergic to the saliva of domestic animals, especially cats, and if they are licked by these animals severe allergy symptoms can occur. The salivary secretions from the family cat are deposited throughout the house. When the saliva dries, it becomes airborne and is inhaled by the allergic child, resulting in a continuing cycle of congestion, cough and possibly asthma. The most positive thing that can be said about animal allergy is that certain breeds of dog or cat may affect some children more than others Patterns of allergic response differ from child to child, and only a little careful sleuthing can establish which animals are likely to produce symptoms and which are not. Sensitivity to an animal does not necessarily mean that pets can never be admitted into the home. But certainly a good deal of guarded control will be necessary if they are.

DIETARY CONTROL

There is no such thing as a completely nonallergenic food; somewhere, sometime, any food you can think of may cause an allergic reaction. Nevertheless, there are more common offenders.

They include:

nuts

dairy products: milk, cheese, cream, etc.

citrus fruits: oranges and grapefruit

cereal grains, primarily wheat

fruits, especially strawberries

sweets, especially chocolate

shellfish, especially prawns and lobster

eggs

By removing a specific food suspected of causing an allergic reaction, you should be able to eliminate the source of the problem. See the chapter on food allergies (p. 208) for a full discussion.

STINGING INSECT CONTROL

Bees and wasps are the most commonly encountered stinging insects. They both belong to the biological order *Hymenoptera* of the class *Insecta*. Hornets are very aggressive and their sting can be dangerous, but they are not common.

Again, avoidance is the key. Wasps tend to sting only if interfered with, and build honeycomb-like nests in trees and places where they are unlikely to be disturbed. Whilst bees are today located mostly in artificial hives, some natural nests can still be found in tree trunks and under floorboards of older houses or other enclosed areas.

Stings from these insects usually produce nothing more serious than a local reaction: a welt or a small swelling. This lesion does not constitute an allergic reaction but is a normal response to toxic substances contained in the insect venom. An allergic reaction occurs when a sting on one area – say, the leg – causes problems in other areas of the body, such as swelling on the arms or the face, hives across the torso, or difficulty in breathing. Severe reactions include significant breathing difficulties, a drop in blood pressure, unconsciousness, shock and, on occasion, death. (There are an average four reported deaths a year caused by allergic insect reactions resulting in anaphylaxis.)

Depending on the allergy, insect-sensitive children should:

Avoid contact with the nest. This of course includes steering clear of beehives, as well as any natural nook and cranny where bees build their hives: the tops of branches, hollow trees, stumps, etc.

Stay away from fields and orchards in flower; these are special haunts of nectar-seeking honeybees.

Avoid gardening. Staying outside for prolonged periods near flowering plants is inviting trouble from honeybees.

Steer clear of areas where organic wastes are stored. Wasps regularly patrol dumps, refuse piles, dustbins and compost heaps.

Not stay outdoors where food is being kept or served. Stinging insects are frequently uninvited visitors to barbecues and picnics.

Not use perfumes, cologne, scented hair tonics and scented deodorants. The odours from all these attract stinging insects. Avoid applying these or any other sweet-smelling potions to your child, especially if much time is being spent outdoors.

Avoid brightly coloured clothing. Strong primary colours, the natural colours of flowers such as greens, yellows and reds, attract many stinging insects. It might be mentioned in passing that mosquitoes are especially fond of the colour blue.

If your child has been diagnosed as being allergic to any of the *Hymenoptera*, keep an *insect sting kit* with you at all times. The older child should be instructed how to use the kit properly. Its contents include antihistamine tablets and a pre-filled syringe containing adrenaline. It is especially useful for allergic children who are entering forested areas or who spend a lot of time outdoors.

PHARMACOTHERAPY

The second of the three main treatment methods used by allergists, pharmacotherapy, involves the use of various oral, injected or inhaled medications. Almost every patient treated for an allergic condition will be given some type of symptomatic medication, and indeed pharmacotherapy is by far the most frequently employed treatment method for the control of allergic symptoms.

Five main categories of drugs are commonly used. At this point a review will help you identify their names and recognize their functions. Later, in the sections on individual allergic ailments, we will take a further look at each of these medicines from the standpoint of specific ailments: how they work, when their prescription is appropriate, what they can and cannot do for the allergic child, possible side effects, and so on down the list of essential considerations. Here are the five categories of drug your child is likely to require.

BRONCHODILATORS

These drugs relax the smooth muscle surrounding the bronchial tubes within the lungs. They are used almost exclusively for the treatment of bronchial asthma.

A number of individual drugs fall under this general heading. The most popular and safe group of drugs are beta-adrenergic agents (beta-agonists). They include salbutamol, terbutaline and fenoterol.

Another group of drugs belong to a group called xanthine derivatives. It includes theophylline and aminophylline. These drugs are older than the beta-adrenergic agents. They are popular with some paediatricians but they have limitations which make chest specialists wary of them. In Australia, the beta-adrenergic drugs are nowadays always preferred to theophylline.

The xanthine and the beta-adrenergic agents work through different pharmacological pathways, but both ultimately bring relief to asthma sufferers in the same way by relaxing and dilating the breathing tubes when they are in spasm.

A third class of bronchodilator drugs are the anti-cholinergic agents. The only one in regular use is ipratropium bromide. They are often used as an adjunct to the beta-adrenergic agents.

SODIUM CROMOGLYCATE

This drug is marketed in a variety of forms. The newest is the Intal inhaler, a metered-dose aerosol spray; it also comes in a capsule form that is inhaled from a device called the Spinhaler. These preparations are used to treat asthma. Rynacrom, a pump-activated nasal spray, is used for allergic rhinitis. Finally there is an ophthalmic form called Opticrom, which is useful for treating allergic conjunctivitis.

Sodium cromoglycate is unique among anti-allergy medi-cines in that its action is prophylactic: it has the ability to block allergic reactions *before* they begin. This means the drugs are helpful only as a preventive measure. If a person is having active symp-toms, sodium cromoglycate will generally be ineffective.

ANTIHISTAMINES

The most familiar of the anti-allergy drugs, antihistamines act to inhibit the action of the chemical substance histamine and are mainly prescribed for the control of perennial and seasonal allergic rhinitis (hay fever). The term antihistamine does not, however, refer to a single drug or even to a particular class of drugs. In actuality there are six different classes of drugs, all of which fall under the antihistamine umbrella.

While most allergic individuals have taken an antihistamine at one time or another, some of the drug's subtle characteristics are not always understood. If, for instance, a certain class of antihistamine does not control your child's symptoms, don't give up, just try another from a different chemical group. This is an especially important point. Somewhere along the line the right preparation will be found, though quite often a trial-and-error approach must be taken before the most effective one is discovered.

Also worth remembering is that if a patient takes an antihistamine from group A and after a month or so the drug loses its effectiveness, a switch to group B antihistamines will often give continued relief. Then, after an appropriate amount of time has elapsed, the patient can return to the original antihistamine from group A and it will once again be effective.

DECONGESTANTS

These drugs help to shrink the swollen mucous membranes of the nose, especially in patients who are suffering from hay fever or animal dander allergies. Unlike many of the antihistamines, decongestants do not cause sleep-producing side-effects, nor will they interfere with the beneficial effects of antihistamines.

A word of warning is in order here concerning over-the-counter nasally administered decongestants: do not take these drugs for more than three to five days at a time. Continued use can lead to the worsening of the very nasal congestion you are trying to control; prolonged use may actually cause irreversible damage to the mucous membranes of the nose. There are more details on this in the section on hay fever (see page 148).

CORTICOSTEROIDS

Cortisone is the best-known example of this potent group of anti-allergic drugs. It is a naturally occurring hormone produced normally by the adrenal glands in response to stress. Extremely useful in treating almost all types of allergic conditions ranging from asthma to itchy rash to chronic nasal problems, cortisone derivatives are available in a variety of forms – creams, ointments, tablets, aerosol sprays, nasal sprays, syrups and injectable solutions.

Except for the weakest-strength creams, the corticosteroid drugs cannot be purchased over the counter and must be prescribed by a doctor. Of all allergy drugs these are perhaps the most powerful *and* the most potentially dangerous. For more concerning their use, see the chapters on asthma, rhinitis, and allergic skin conditions.

EXPECTORANTS

Many allergic patients suffer from a chronic cough that produces a thick, sticky mucus that is difficult to cough up and spit out. Expectorant drugs, at least in theory, work on these secretions, helping to keep them in a more fluid state and allowing the patient to expel them with greater ease. Expectorants can be purchased over the counter at any chemist, though in my opinion, fluids of any kind – especially plain water, hot or cold – are as good as most of the commercial preparations available today.

PHYSIOTHERAPY AND EXERCISE

Physical therapy is an important adjunct to the overall care of allergic children in general and asthmatic children in particular. Techniques can take the form of a specific set of breathing exercises taught to the child by a physiotherapist, or they may involve a more general plan of participation in games and athletics.

As a rule, all allergic and especially asthmatic children should be encouraged to participate in physical activities appropriate to their age group and physical condition. Preventing a child with an allergic problem from becoming involved in normal play creates both a bad self-image and unavoidable conflict with other children. There are few more pathetic sights than that of a schoolchild sitting sullenly on the playground bench, passively watching friends romp during break or in gym. Such a child quickly turns into the class outcast or invalid, and other children are rarely shy about rubbing it in.

Of course, physical activity in some children may cause the very symptoms you are trying to avoid, but there are almost always medications which keep these symptoms under control and which allow the child to play as children must. Activities which demand constant running such as football or rugby are more likely than others to trigger wheezing attacks, and the severely asthmatic child should probably steer clear of them. Other sports such as swimming, tennis, cricket and cycling are in general quite well tolerated and in many cases have a therapeutic effect on the child. Encourage them.

Finally, for children who suffer from bronchial asthma, an adjunct therapy frequently recommended is an exercise called diaphragmatic breathing. This interesting technique teaches the child to use his diaphragm in such a way that deeper, more relaxed and effective breaths are taken; this helps to raise mucus secretions more easily from the lower parts of the bronchial tubes. I provide a specific exercise for diaphragmatic breathing (Belly Breathing) in the Appendix. Essentially, breathing exercises provide a relaxing diversion for the child with asthma. They will enable the youngster to control asthma symptoms better during an attack.

HYPOSENSITIZATION OR DESENSITIZATION

The last form of allergy therapy is known as desensitization or immunotherapy and until recently was the treatment most people associated with visiting an allergist. Following skin testing or, in the case of hay fever, when the occurrence of symptoms at a particular time of year was so characteristic that skin testing was not needed, a series of injections of the particular allergen were given. Treatment was started with very low doses of the allergens; if the injections were well tolerated the dose was increased in a controlled fashion up to a maintenance dose level. Various regimes were used, the most popular being a course of weekly injections over two to three months and then, if a maintenance dose was considered necessary, injections every month or so. These courses could be repeated in successive years with the doses changed slightly to take into account changing sensitivity.

These courses were never very popular with young children because of the necessity of repeated injections for relatively mild symptoms. However, teenagers and adults were treated for hay fever and house dust mite allergies regularly with varying success.

Asthma was usually found not to be a suitable candidate for this sort of treatment, as the usual strength of the starting doses tended to precipitate quite severe attacks. Even if special dilutions were used with the doses taken down to minute levels, dangerous reactions still occurred and in many cases the procedure had to be abandoned.

However, in 1986 the UK Committee on Safety of Medicines recommended restriction in the use of hyposensitizing vaccines because of the reports of a number of deaths from acute anaphylaxis. The restrictions were so stringent that the injection could be given only with the back-up facilities which are usually only found in major hospitals; a two-hour wait after each injection was also advised. Because of these restrictions the practice of hyposensitization has almost come to a standstill. The one exception is the vaccines given for allergy to bee and wasp stings. The allergies themselves can be so dangerous that the risks inherent in hyposensitization are reasonable and there is no other adequate way of protecting those involved.

TREATING THE TREATED CHILD

In any situation where a child has chronic or recurring symptoms and is receiving special treatment, parental support and constant encouragement play a very important role in the overall management approach. Fortunately, most allergic conditions are not very severe and are more of an annoyance – significant at times – than a major problem. Still, such support is a crucial part of the therapy itself.

The best steps parents can take, after making sure that their child is treated by a competent doctor and that the household environment is friendly to allergy-free living, is to be appropriately concerned when an attack occurs, to empathize as fully as possible with the child's psychological situation and, above all, to remember what sickness of any kind was like for oneself as a child. Parents must also steer a narrow course between, on the one hand, overcoddling children when trouble starts and, on the other, becoming gradually callous and unresponsive to their complaints.

Perhaps the most important of all virtues when dealing with an allergic child is sympathy tempered by common sense.

In some instances, of course, the situation is more demanding, as with severe asthma or eczema. In such cases there is almost certain to be dramatic impact on the life of the entire family. Depending on the age and temperament of the child, the handling of this situation must be different in different cases. No matter what approach is taken, however, it is of the greatest importance that the child be made to understand that he can and *must* lead as nearly normal a life as possible.

This means that overprotecting children or continually reminding them how sick they are is an instinct to avoid. If you are going to err, do so on the side of permissiveness in matters such as participation in sports or vigorous activities, in allowing the child to hike, fish, camp and run free like other children. One of the more serious mistakes parents can make is to act as though their child were different – handicapped, crippled or odd – incapable of doing the things that other children do. The more a youngster is urged to participate in usual childhood activities, the less likely she will consider herself to be abnormal or different. The importance of providing a seriously allergic child with a strong, positive self-image cannot be overstressed.

QUESTIONS AND ANSWERS ABOUT ALLERGIES AND ALLERGISTS

How can I tell if an allergist is competent?

Take the advice of your GP, who will know and have worked with the local allergists and will be aware of their experience. Allergists usually have the general postgraduate qualification of Member of the Royal College of Physicians (MRCP), after which they specialize in allergy. As yet they have no unique postgraduate body, although there are moves afoot to that end.

What is the best way to handle a child who is afraid of visiting an allergist?

As usual, honesty is the best policy with children. If your child is particularly uneasy about the forthcoming visit, it is your responsibility to gather as much preparatory information as possible. This may require a phone call, either to the consultant's secretary-receptionist or even to the consultant himself concerning what will take place at the visit. This information should then be passed on to your child simply and directly. If your child continues to fear the visit, inform the consultant about it beforehand to allow planning the examination and testing procedures accordingly.

What are some of the specific things you can tell children to relieve them of fear?

Probably the thing children fear most about a visit to the allergist is getting a 'jab'. Since the time injections first became a standard part of medical procedure, stories have circulated among children about needles at the doctor's, some of which, no doubt, measure a foot long or maybe even two! Just the word 'jab' itself conjures up images of impact and pain.

From my experience the only way to remove a child's anxiety on this subject is to have the doctor carefully explain beforehand exactly what he is and is not going to do. He must approach this task in a relaxed, unhurried and sympathetic manner. Quite often I will do the first test on the parent so that the child can be an observer before becoming a participant.

In many cases the expectations of parents concerning a visit to the allergist can be so great to the child that they unwittingly convey either a sense of anxiety or an unrealistic anticipation of a 'total cure'. Neither is desirable. Simply tell the child that he will soon be visiting a doctor who has a particular interest in his allergy problem and who wants to find out what causes it, and to help it. Respond to all questions with simple, clear answers. Never evade a question, but don't get too technical, either. Be honest: if you know that a test is going to be done, and that it involves a particular procedure, say so.

The fact is that some children who visit an allergist have had previous exposure to allergy testing. If parents learn about these tests before coming to the consulting room, if they discuss them with their child with assurance and honesty, if the doctor is not rushed or abrupt when administering them, and if time is taken at the initial visit to establish the all-important doctor–parent–patient relationship, the whole evaluation will prove a positive experience.

What is the best way to prepare a child for a long-term series of treatments?

With the almost complete cessation of desensitization for hay fever, etc. – this procedure being reserved for more serious bee and wasp sting allergies – this situation will rarely crop up nowadays. The tests and treatments are neither frightening nor painful.

Is it wise for a doctor to talk about a child's condition in front of the child?

I feel a child should be involved in all discussions regarding her allergic condition. There are only very rare exceptions to this policy. Education of the entire family is one of the major contributions the doctor can provide, and the more everyone knows about the specific problem, the better the outcome will be for the patient. Children can assume much more responsibility for their own medical management than they have been given credit for.

How long will the first visit usually take?

This varies from doctor to doctor. An average consultation probably takes about an hour.

How expensive will it be?

First of all, it need not cost you anything. If your GP refers you, you can have all the necessary treatment on the NHS. If you wish to go privately, again, if your referral is sanctioned by your GP, your fees should be reimbursable from private medical insurance. The one proviso is that you have been insured since before the condition started. If, on going on a private medical insurance scheme, you were asked if there were any pre-existing medical condition and allergy was mentioned, there may be a clause in your contract which excludes allergy. If you have only just joined a scheme and have not mentioned pre-existing allergy, remember that your GP will have to fill in a form giving the date of the first consultation *by any doctor* for this condition, before you get reimbursed. So if in doubt about your eligibility for benefit, check with your insurers.

If you are not insured, there is no reason why you cannot ask a private allergist what his fees will be before embarking on a potentially expensive and prolonged course of treatment, as private consultants' fees will vary from doctor to doctor and in different parts of the country. Forewarned is forearmed.

What if you cannot get a quote of fees by phone?

You then have a perfectly understandable reason for bypassing the doctor and going to the next. Usually there should be no difficulty in getting a prior quote for the fees.

Can allergic symptoms change? For example, can an allergic skin condition become a nasal problem? Or a chest problem?

In some cases, yes. The development of allergic symptomatology is sometimes progressive. For example, quite often a young child will develop an allergic skin condition that disappears within twelve to twenty-four months. Once the skin problem vanishes, however, symptoms of allergic rhinitis or asthma may replace it. (This relationship between allergic skin conditions and nasal or chest symptoms has been called the dermal-respiratory syndrome.) There is no set pattern to the way these symptoms shift.

If allergic symptoms are neglected, will they worsen?

If symptoms are caused by exposure to a specific allergen and the child is constantly exposed to this substance without being treated, the symptoms will probably become more serious.

But there are other considerations, too. If a child has an itchy rash and the parents do nothing to control it, the itching sensation will almost certainly worsen. Because of persistent scratching the rash will spread and there is a good chance that it will become secondarily infected. Common sense would suggest that an ounce of prevention provided by early medical treatment will be worth more than a pound of cure afterwards.

Similarly, if a child suffers from allergic nasal symptoms and nothing is done to control them, the ailment will not necessarily become worse. But it *will* persist and it *will* become chronic and it *will* invite all the secondary woes such a chronic condition can bring: permanently chapped upper lip, red nose, itchy eyes, the exhaustion of incessant sneezing, and so on. Again, preventive medicine is the wisest course. Early medical treatment is clearly the best way – and really the only way – to treat an allergic symptom.

Certain allergic ailments – asthma in particular – unequivocally call for medical treatment right away, now, immediately and without delay. To assume that a laboured breathing is not a serious enough reason to warrant a trip to the doctor, or that the problem will go away on its own when the child gets older, is to look for trouble. Furthermore, one should not assume that after an asthmatic attack is over the child will never have a recurrence. Once the first asthma attack occurs, there is a good chance that other episodes will develop.

In essence then, parents are well advised to do *something* about allergic symptoms, even if it is only using over-the-counter medications to achieve temporary relief. In most cases symptoms will get progressively worse without treatment. At best they will stay the same; and this is no pleasure for the child.

Are there any cases where medication is not necessary?

Lesley is five years old. She lives across the street from a friendly older widow who owns three friendly old cats. Whenever Lesley visits the woman and her pets – or when she visits anyone who happens to own cats – the dander from the animals makes her sneeze.

Several hours after leaving the woman's house Lesley's symptoms vanish and they don't start up again until her next visit. Lesley's allergic reaction is relatively mild, and the pleasure she derives from playing with the animals, in her parents' estimation (and also, by the way, in her own), outweighs the temporary discomfort the contact brings. In such a case, when the allergen is native to a particular place and can normally be avoided, when the symptoms disappear quickly, and when the symptoms themselves are minor, then medication is not necessary.

Do children outgrow allergies?

Sometimes. While we are not certain what the term 'outgrow' really means, we do know that over a period of time many children show a decrease in allergic symptoms, both in frequency and intensity. This does *not* hold true for everybody, specifically in the case of asthma. If we take a hundred five-year-old asthmatic children and observe them for a ten-year period, we will see that approximately a third of these children have no obvious asthma symptoms at ages ten to fifteen, that a third have remained the same, and that a third have got worse. Can we identify which child will fall into which of these categories? No. It's impossible for a doctor to look at a five-year-old and say, 'You're going to get better' or 'You're going to get worse'.

At the same time, some facts can assist the doctor in making what amounts to an educated guess. Family history of asthma, the course of the asthma condition since its start, and the patient's response to medication can sometimes suggest what direction the child's condition will take.

So one should never assume that with the passage of time children will automatically shed their allergies?

The chances are roughly one in three that they will. The situation can be illusive, too, as allergies sometimes go into a kind of remission during adolescence, only to reappear years later. Again, this is particularly true in the case of asthma. Bear in mind that there is nothing magical about the period of puberty which parents of allergic children await with such great anticipation. While many physical and hormonal changes do occur at this time, nature by no means guarantees that a reduction of allergic response will be one of them. Some children get better; some get worse. It's one of nature's many unfathomable lotteries.

Some parents assume that their child has outgrown a serious hay fever or bothersome skin condition when in fact she has simply been removed from its cause. If a child lives in the country then moves to the city and the next year ceases to have attacks, this does not necessarily constitute a cure. To be fully sure that the child has 'outgrown' a sensitivity, the child must return to the source of the allergen and continue to remain symptom-free.

Will childhood allergies ever disappear spontaneously, on their own?

Occasionally, but only occasionally, so don't bank on it. Better to work from the premise that the allergy will *not* disappear on its own; and then, if it happens to do so, give thanks that your child is among the fortunate few.

Are childhood allergies more common in one sex than in the other?

In early childhood, boys develop allergic symptoms more frequently than girls. During adolescence the graph reverses, and females statistically become more vulnerable. No one knows exactly why.

Can an allergic condition severely cripple or disable a child?

One day a five-year-old girl came into my consulting room with a case of eczema so advanced that she was hardly able to walk. The creases behind her knees had become badly infected and it was almost impossible for her to bend her legs; she had to be carried into the examining room.

So the answer is yes, a child can be severely handicapped by an allergic disease, and this does not just include the most obvious instance of respiratory crippling that takes place in untreated asthma. Severe sneezing and weeping eyes during the hay fever season can, for instance, become so debilitating that the child ceases to function normally and may not be able to attend school. Most cases of this kind, it should be added, develop in children who have *not* been cared for by a doctor in the early stages.

What is the most severe form of allergic reaction a child can develop?

It is known as anaphylaxis, a generalized reaction involving the skin, respiratory and cardiovascular systems. An allergic child can develop anaphylaxis from exposure to any allergen to which he is sensitive. Symptoms consist of any one or all of the following: a generalized itchy rash (urticaria or hives), shortness of breath, tightness of the chest, wheezing (asthma), drop in blood pressure (hypotension) and loss of consciousness (syncope). Anaphylaxis is frequently associated with allergic reactions to foods, drugs, and insect stings. A true medical emergency, it calls for the *immediate* attention of a doctor. If untreated, it may ultimately prove fatal. With prompt medical treatment an anaphylactic reaction can be successfully controlled.

Under what circumstances can an allergic condition be fatal?

In certain rare cases. As I've said, an anaphylactic reaction, if untreated, has the potential to end in death. Also, a severe asthma attack can clog the breathing passages with thick mucus plugs and suffocate the patient. It is estimated that, in the UK, around 1,500 people a year die from asthma, approximately 2 per cent of them children. On average, four people per year die from allergic reactions to bee or wasp stings.

Can a child who has not been treated for an allergy in its early stages recover sufficiently in the hands of a competent allergist if treated at a later date?

As a rule, the proper identification and avoidance of specific allergic substances, along with the use of appropriate medications, can transform most children from passive observers of life into active participants. A new patient of mine was prevented from participating in her favourite sports because of a severe asthmatic condition. After being started on a proper management programme with an appropriate bronchodilator drug, she quickly took up athletics again and eventually became the star of her volleyball team. The moral of this story and many others like it is that even the most severely asthmatic child can be significantly helped.

Will a run-down or sickly child be more likely to develop allergies than a healthy one?

There is at present no medical evidence to indicate that a debilitated child runs an increased risk of developing allergic symptoms. The causes of allergy seem to have almost exclusively genetic, cellular and environmental origins.

Is there an average age at which allergies begin to develop in children?

While the age of onset generally spans the spectrum of the childhood years, there is a tendency for certain conditions, specifically eczema and food allergies, to occur during the first years or even the first months of life. Problems such as hay fever tend to begin after the child is three or four. Asthma can develop at any time, from infancy to adolescence. Sensitivities to substances such as antibiotics, aspirin, insect stings and environmental pollutants can develop at almost any age.

Can a newborn child be allergic?

While it is theoretically possible for a newborn baby to become sensitized in utero and therefore respond allergically, such cases are quite unusual. I can, however, recall seeing a three-day-old infant develop allergic nasal congestion from drinking a milk-based formula. Other infants not infrequently develop intestinal symptoms such as diarrhoea and vomiting after being fed a milk-based formula. I have also seen very young children develop eczema because of a food allergy.

How long does it usually take for an allergic reaction to appear once a child has made contact with an allergen?

It depends on the child's degree of sensitivity. In some situations the reactions will begin almost immediately after contact, particularly if the young person happens to be highly susceptible.

Allergic symptoms can develop very rapidly or can evolve gradually over a period of hours following exposure to a specific allergen.

Are allergies ever contagious?

No, never. Allergic children sometimes develop a nasty-sounding cough mistakenly labelled bronchitis. The youngster is then sent home or kept out of school for no reason other than misdiagnosis. As a doctor I am constantly writing notes to teachers, explaining that even though Johnny is sneezing his head off or coughing violently the problem is an allergic one, not an infectious one, and that it poses no threat to other children.

Part Two

The Treatment of Specific Allergic Conditions

CHAPTER FIVE

Asthma

First the bad news: while we can't give exact numbers, it is estimated that approximately 5 per cent of the UK population today suffer from some form of bronchial asthma. Of this group, approximately 1,500 will die each year directly from the disease. In Australia and New Zealand, one in five children between the ages of five and nine suffer from some sort of asthma attack. Fortunately, the number of asthma fatalities occurring in children represents only a very, very small percentage of this figure! Another group, no one knows how large, will suffer from ailments to which it is a contributing cause. Among children, millions of school days will be lost each year because of asthma, and in many paediatric wards it will be one of the two or three most common ailments for which children are admitted. Indeed, concern for an asthmatic child will sometimes become so total that it dominates all aspects of family life, from holiday planning to the daily menu; every decision must eventually hinge on the inevitable question of whether it will conflict with Susie's 'condition'. So don't be fooled: asthma can be a serious matter. The cost in terms of time and money, disruption of family life and plain human suffering is impossible to calculate. It is not a condition to be minimized and certainly not one to be ignored.

On the other hand – and here's the good news – despite the many potential problems, the overwhelming majority of children with asthma can function normally. Their symptoms can be so well controlled that they will live active, healthy lives.

While asthma has been recognized as a medical condition since the time of Hippocrates, it is still difficult to come up with a definition that is accepted by all doctors. The ailment seems to be triggered by so many diverse agents, the symptoms can differ so widely among sufferers, and the actual cause of the sickness is still not completely understood, so a definition on which everyone agrees continues to elude us.

Such lack of unanimity notwithstanding, the following simple definition covers most of the important aspects of this disorder and will serve adequately for our purposes.

Asthma is a reversible, obstructive airways disease.

Let's take a close look at this sentence.

Asthma is reversible. This means that almost always the severe breathing difficulties that occur during an asthma attack can, with proper treatment, be reversed to normal breathing patterns and that permanent lung damage does not result from such attacks, even in the worst cases.

These are comforting facts for parents to recognize: *the symptoms of asthma are not permanent*, and *with proper treatment* they can *be reversed to a normal condition.* A diagnosis of asthma is by no means a sentence of doom or banishment from childhood fun. Today there are many professional and Olympic-class athletes who suffered with bronchial asthma as children, many opera singers, many ballet dancers, marathon runners and heavy-duty labourers, all of whom live normal lives today, their asthma kept well controlled by effective and appropriate medication.

Asthma is an obstructive condition. A child wheezes because the air passageways (bronchial tubes) are obstructed and therefore air cannot be easily expelled from the lungs. This obstruction is caused by three factors:

When an attack begins, the smooth muscles surrounding the breathing tubes (bronchi) go into spasm and tighten, thereby narrowing the bronchi.

When stimulated during an attack, the mucus glands lining the breathing passageways produce large amounts of very thick, sticky mucus (normal mucus is thin and watery in consistency). These increased secretions can block the smallest air passageways (respiratory bronchioles) and worsen the asthma attack.

Finally, because of inflammation and irritation within the

smallest breathing passageways, several things occur: there is swelling of the cells lining the bronchioles (the smallest bronchi) and a build-up of cellular debris from dead tissue cells, viruses and bacteria. The end result is a significant decrease in the size of the bronchial airways.

These three interdependent processes produce a wide range of physical symptoms. These include:

tightness in the chest

shortness of breath

fatigue

coughing

wheezing

anxiety

most conspicuously, an inability to catch one's breath

It should be added that not every patient has all these symptoms during every attack. Still, everyone who experiences a mild asthma attack is aware that something decidedly unpleasant is taking place and that the lungs are by no means functioning as they should.

Asthma is a disease of the airways. It is in the bronchial tubes that the asthmatic process takes place. The disease is *not* centred in the air sacs whose job it is to take oxygen to the body and transport carbon dioxide for removal from the body. Asthma is strictly a disease of the breathing passageways.

Note that the word *allergy* does not appear in our definition, and for good reason: a child need not suffer from allergies to have asthma. His asthma may be triggered by either allergic or nonallergic causes.

Nonallergic asthma Originally termed 'intrinsic asthma' because there were no obvious external causes. It was believed that the reason for the attack came from something *within* the person. Today it is recognized that there are many nonallergic triggers for asthma. A partial list includes: viral respiratory infections, changing

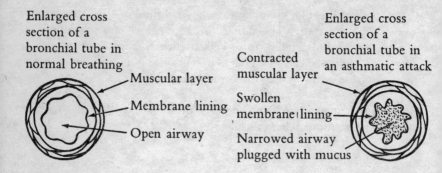

Enlarged cross section of a bronchial tube in normal breathing

Muscular layer

Membrane lining

Open airway

Contracted muscular layer

Enlarged cross section of a bronchial tube in an asthmatic attack

Swollen membrane lining

Narrowed airway plugged with mucus

Figure 1 The anatomy of asthma

SOURCE: National Heart, Lung, and Blood Institute, USA

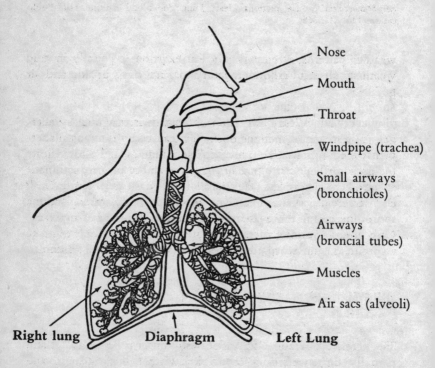

Nose

Mouth

Throat

Windpipe (trachea)

Small airways (bronchioles)

Airways (broncial tubes)

Muscles

Air sacs (alveoli)

Right lung   **Diaphragm**   **Left Lung**

Figure 2(a) Normal lungs

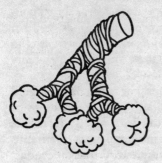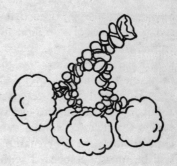

Figure 2(b) Inside the lungs during an asthma attack

CREDIT: National Heart, Lung, & Blood Institute, USA
SOURCE: C. H. Feldman and N. M. Clark, *Open Airways/Respiro Abierto: Asthma Self-Management Program*, National Heart, Lung, and Blood Institute, NIH Publications No. 84–2365.

weather patterns, strenuous physical exertion (especially in cold weather), stressful emotional situations, irritating odours and air pollution.

Allergic asthma Allergic, or 'external' asthma is triggered by allergens originating outside the body. It is caused by the typical allergens we have met so far – dust, pollen, dander, etc. To complicate the issue further, many patients have the ability to react asthmatically to both types of stimuli, the allergic and the nonallergic. Such children are diagnosed as having a 'mixed' form of asthma. Asthma symptoms are the same regardless of the specific cause of an attack. Only after a complete allergy evaluation will it be possible to make a specific diagnosis regarding the cause(s) of your child's asthma.

THE SYMPTOMS OF ASTHMA: WHAT TO LOOK FOR AND WHAT TO IGNORE

The perennial question 'Why does my child have asthma?' is still partially unanswerable. We do know that both genetic and environmental factors play a role, and that children with asthma have 'hyperactive airways' (some refer to them as 'twitchy lungs').

Such supersensitive bronchial passageways are especially responsive to a variety of stimuli including allergens (dust, foods, pollens, animal danders, etc.), physical exertion, viral infections and emotional stress. Exposure to any of these triggers can rapidly bring on an attack.

Bronchial hyper-reactivity is thus the one physiological abnormality common to everyone with asthma. The situations or events that trigger asthma symptoms can vary greatly from one child to the next. For example, for some youngsters symptoms will be mostly associated with upper respiratory tract infections. Every time the child has a mild cold, an asthma attack will develop. Others show a clear pattern of asthma only at specific times of year. These children sometimes develop asthma secondary to reactions to mould spores or to specific pollens which are airborne during certain months, especially in the spring and autumn. For yet another group of children, foods may be the triggering mechanism. For still others animal dander or feathers are the culprits.

Other causes of asthma? Take your pick: strenuous physical exercise; dampness or cold; cigarette smoke; extremely dusty environments; irritating odours; excessive laughter; strong winds; household chemicals; air pollution – the list goes on. For some patients only a few of these agents will cause problems. For others a panoply of potential asthma triggers lurk both in nature and around the house. And for a small minority of unfortunate individuals all the situations mentioned above, as well as others yet unlisted, can catapult them into a full-blown asthmatic attack.

Merely labelling a child as asthmatic doesn't say very much. As a doctor I have seen children who wheeze only rarely, who have no trouble breathing, and who in fact show no other respiratory symptoms. Yet, clinically speaking, these children have bronchial asthma. At the other end of the spectrum, I have cared for children who in spite of all the effective anti-asthma medicines available continue to wheeze and struggle for breath every day of their lives.

There is no single clinical pattern for the young patient with asthma. I constantly find myself telling parents of asthmatic children that the one consistent thing about asthma is its inconsistency. If you are the parent of an asthmatic child, it is important to keep this point in mind: the pattern of asthma symptoms in this child and the pattern of symptoms in that child will not necessarily –

and probably won't – be the same as the pattern of symptoms in *your* child.

Having said all this, here is a list of the possible symptoms that alone or together should heighten suspicion that your child may have asthma:

wheezing, noted primarily when breathing out (expiration)

complaints of tightness in the chest

an inability to take a deep breath

an inability to breathe comfortably while lying down

complaints of chest and stomach pains

a constant harsh cough

If any combination of these symptoms continues for more than twelve to twenty-four hours, consult your doctor. At any time you feel your child's symptoms are obviously worsening, get some medical assistance either by telephone or a visit to the surgery.

There are additional points to bear in mind about identifying asthma symptomatology. Between attacks there are usually no abnormal physical findings when a child is examined by a doctor. The symptoms of asthma can stay unusually well hidden until the hour of attack. It will often take special tests and equipment to detect respiratory abnormalities of any kind during symptom-free times.

Andy, aged ten, wheezes once or twice a year. Chris, who is eleven, has shortness of breath and a sensation of chest tightness several times a week. Here are two patients with bronchial asthma, and neither considers himself to be 'sick'. In Andy's case the conclusion is understandable. Chris's reaction is more surprising, perhaps, but it is also refreshingly healthy. The point is that most children with chronic asthma symptoms will wish to ignore their symptoms and get on with their lives. When such an attitude begins to emerge, parents are well advised to co-operate fully. In all but the most severe cases, asthmatic children should be encouraged to participate in a full range of social and athletic activities, and parents of these children should under no circumstances hold them back with ominous warnings about 'strain' or 'overdoing'. In fact, it is an axiom: the less the asthma bothers the child, the less it should bother the parent.

If a child is old enough to have pulmonary function (breathing) studies done, most patients will show *some* detectable abnormalities of lung function. Even when the child displays no manifest symptoms, pulmonary function test abnormalities can show up. This is true even many years after a person has had his last attack. The true significance of this finding is not understood. An abnormal pulmonary function study may possibly indicate a poor prognosis later on in life. The final answer on this question is still up in the air.

During an attack, wheezing, noted mainly though not exclusively when exhaling, is *the* most common symptom of asthma and is by and large the hallmark of the disease. If your child starts to have periods of respiratory discomfort, and if these attacks are accompanied by audible wheezing sounds, place asthma high on the list of possible disorders.

During an asthma attack, a patient's respiratory rate – the number of respirations she takes per minute – will increase as the hours pass. At the same time, the depth of breathing – that is, the ability to take a full breath – will *decrease*. This is another indication that an attack is worsening.

During an asthma attack, bronchospasm and narrowing of the airways make it progressively more difficult for the child to exhale (usually inhaling is not a problem). Because of progressively worsening bronchial obstruction air becomes 'trapped' in the balloon-like air sacs, which eventually causes the lungs to swell and the chest to expand. Children who suffer from severe and continual asthmatic episodes sometimes develop a chest abnormality known as 'pigeon breast deformity'. (If you can picture a pigeon with its chest puffed out, you can visualize how the chest of a severely asthmatic child may sometimes appear.)

Parents will find that children commonly suffer from asthma attacks at night. This may result from the fact that lying in a horizontal sleeping position causes mucous secretions to accumulate in the lungs. Or it may be due to the decreased production of cortisone in the child's system while he is asleep. Whatever the case, if your child is having problems with nocturnal attacks it is a good idea always to have the proper medications on hand *before* local chemist's shops close down for the evening.

RECOGNIZING AND ASSESSING AN ASTHMA EMERGENCY

At the beginning of any attack, notice that your child is breathing mainly by means of the chest muscles. As the attack progresses and as breathing becomes more laboured, both the abdominal and the upper chest and neck muscles may join in the process, and eventually the space between the ribs, the bottom of the ribcage, and the area above the collarbones will all appear to be sucked in with every breath. These movements of the thorax are called 'retractions' and are an indication that the patient's respiratory distress is increasing. When retractions are noted, which means the child is working harder to breathe, it is time to contact your doctor.

Many children, especially younger ones, also complain of abdominal distress during asthma attacks. The problem develops for several reasons. First, due to downward pressure of the diaphragm caused by air trapped in the lungs, the stomach is squeezed in an unaccustomed manner, in some cases causing a severe stomach ache. Second, many young children swallow excessive amounts of air during an attack; the stomach becomes accordingly distended and exerts pressure on the nerves, which in turn produce sharp abdominal pains. Though the child may be in acute misery from these cramps, they are rarely dangerous. However, do not ignore these symptoms. Third, many children swallow large amounts of mucus during an attack, which in turn produce significant abdominal irritation. As the asthma symptoms are brought under control, all these abdominal complaints will slowly subside.

During an attack, a child's heart and lungs work extraordinarily hard. As a result, heart rate is greatly accelerated. A rapid pulse does not usually mean trouble and is in fact to be expected whenever increased demands are made on the cardiac and respiratory systems. Consider what takes place after a session of intense physical activity – our hearts pound, breathing is rapid, the body sweats — and all these reactions are, of course, perfectly normal. You should realize that your child is experiencing the same physical sensations during an attack. Rarely, if ever, are cardiac problems or heart damage associated with such activity. Your child's pulse and respiratory rate will return to normal once the acute attack is brought under control.

If an attack is prolonged and no treatment is forthcoming, the child may begin to wheeze *less* than at the start of the episode. This situation generally takes many hours or even several days to develop. When it does occur — and if there is no corresponding ease of breathing to signify that the attack itself is subsiding — it is a serious warning sign. Repeat: *it is not a good sign.* If the chest becomes 'silent', this is because the bronchial air passageways are now so clogged with thickened, gluelike mucus that little or no air is moving through the lungs. The child's lungs are receiving inadequate amounts of air: hence not enough oxygen is reaching the bloodstream. The process, in short, is a prelude to suffocation.

If the 'silent' chest syndrome continues without treatment, or if the air passageways remain blocked for extensive periods of time, the child may also show signs of cyanosis, or lack of oxygen. Clinically, this condition can be recognized when the lips and fingernail beds turn bluish. The nail beds at the base of your child's fingernails are normally a lively pinkish-white. During a severe asthmatic attack, lack of oxygen to the lungs turns them a morbid shade of blue, an indication that the attack is reaching the critical point.

Cyanosis requires *immediate* medical attention. REPEAT: IMMEDIATE! If your doctor is not available, get to the nearest hospital casualty department without delay. The situation has reached the emergency stage. Suffocation is beginning.

During an asthma attack a child's rate of breathing will inevitably increase, and with each breath a measurable loss of water vapour follows. Children, especially very young ones, usually cannot tolerate eating or drinking during an attack, and these two factors — the loss of water vapour and the refusal or inability to take solids and liquids — frequently result in dehydration.

Loss of water from the lungs then causes mucus in the bronchi to become thick and gluelike, producing added blockage

SIX SIGNS THAT SUGGEST A TRIP TO THE DOCTOR*

wheezing gets worse one to three hours after taking medicine

child stops playing and cannot start again

child has hard time breathing

breathing gets faster one to three hours after taking medicine

child has trouble walking or talking

blue lips or fingernails – go immediately!

*SOURCE: C. H. Feldman and N. M. Clark, *Open Airways/Respiro Abierto: Asthma Self-Management Program*, National Heart, Lung, and Blood Institute, NIH Publication No. 84–2365.

of the airways and hence increased respiratory discomfort. It is therefore vitally important that children be made to take some liquids during an attack, even though eating and drinking are the farthest things from their minds, and that this be done by whatever methods are at hand. Don't be reluctant to offer soda, lemonade, water, anything wet. Some children like to suck on cracked ice. Other prefer warm liquids through a straw. Whatever you do, make sure that moderate amounts of fluids get *in*. If signs of dehydration are already present (symptoms include dry tongue, decrease in urination and a loss of the elastic quality of the skin), the child should receive immediate medical care.

There is a series of relatively simple medical observations that you as a parent can make to assess the seriousness of your child's condition.

● Check respiration rates. How many breaths per minute are being taken? Using a watch, count the number of inhalations registered in thirty seconds. Double this number and you have the breaths-per-minute count. A normal rate, generally speaking, should be under twenty-four inhalations per minute (infants, as a rule, breathe somewhat faster – up to thirty breaths a minute). Each child's respiratory rate differs slightly, of course, so I suggest you determine this figure during an asthma-free period. Approach children while they are reading or watching TV, and record the number of breaths taken in a thirty-second stretch (count the inhalation and exhalation as one complete breath). Then file this figure away for future reference. Measure it against your child's normal repiratory rate during the next asthmatic episode.

When does an increased breath count become cause for alarm? It is safe to say that more than thirty to thirty-five breaths per minute is increased. If this number climbs above forty per minute, the danger zone has been entered: the child is obviously having respiratory distress and is working very hard to breathe. Seek medical help at once.

● Check the pulse rate. How fast is the heart beating? The easiest pulses to count are located on the thumb side of the wrist (radial pulse) and along either side of the neck (carotid pulse). During an attack the neck vessels become especially prominent – you can sometimes see them throbbing – and are easy to locate. Count the number of beats at either of these pulse points for fifteen seconds, multiply this number by four, and you have the pulse-per-minute rate.

A healthy and/or dangerous pulse rate differs for children according to their age, and again, infants have higher counts than older children. Pulse rates, in general, approach the danger zone when they climb above 120. If the count exceeds 125, talk to your doctor. It is also a good idea to keep a record of your child's resting pulse and respiration rate handy, even during asthma-free times. These statistics will help your doctor to gain a clear picture of the child's condition at your next visit. They can also be used as a baseline against which to gauge the seriousness of an attack when it occurs at home.

● Each time your child has a substantial bout of asthma, check carefully for retractions. Retractions are sucking-in motions of the soft tissues located between, over and under the ribcage. Look carefully for them in the area above the collarbone. Are the movements confined to the abdominal and chest area? Your doctor will want to know precisely where the retractions are located and how long they have been present.

• Observe the nature of your child's cough. Though the noise of a loose rattle and associated mucus build-up may sound unpleasant, this very loose, loud quality is probably a positive sign. It is the body's method of clearing foreign matter out of the bronchial tree and moving mucus secretions from one area of the lung to another until they can be coughed out or swallowed. When mucus is expectorated, moreover, its colour and texture offer critical clues to what is taking place in the lungs. Thin, clear and whitish mucus is, generally speaking, a good sign. Mucus that is discoloured or coughed up in firm plugs indicates that an infection may be present or an attack has been going on for a fairly long time.

If the nature of the child's cough changes from loose and wet to persistent, dry and hacking, this means the attack is worsening. Speak to the doctor right away.

• Is your child able to retain food, fluids and medication? If not, be aware that nausea and vomiting may occur. For a number of reasons, it is always important to determine the cause and be able to control these symptoms.

Young children will frequently vomit as a result of having swallowed large amounts of mucus, a substance highly irritating to the lining of the stomach. They may also develop this symptom when the stomach becomes distended and swollen with large amounts of swallowed air. Downward pressure of the diaphragm on the stomach is another possible explanation for vomiting.

The bronchodilator medications used to control the asthma attack can sometimes trigger vomiting, either because of gastric irritation or as a toxic symptom of theophylline overdosage.

As a rule, during an attack children feel better after they have vomited the large amounts of irritating mucus which accumulate in the stomach. However, if the vomiting continues, call the doctor. Be prepared to tell him how frequently the child has vomited and to describe the regurgitated material.

Never allow an attack of asthma to go on too long before consulting a doctor. And don't suppose that this particular episode will be shorter than the last: there is no reason to make such an assumption; the opposite can just as easily be true. Remember, *the longer an asthmatic attack is allowed to continue without treatment, the more difficult it will be to control once medical advice is sought.* Get help early, before things get worse.

SOME SIGNIFICANT FACTS YOU SHOULD KNOW ABOUT ASTHMA

Asthma and the emotions Despite a lingering popular notion that asthma is an 'emotional disease', instances of asthma originating exclusively or even primarily in psychological causes are, in my experience, unusual. This is not to suggest that a child who experiences recurrent asthmatic episodes may not develop an emotional response to the condition, or that stressful psychological situations do not occasionally worsen the disease. Such emotional or psychological reactions are, however, *secondary* to the underlying condition itself. They are, so to speak, side effects and are rarely the actual cause of the attack. According to what is known today, asthma is first and foremost a physiological disorder. It is *not* the result of an emotional disorder. All the more reason for parents to be aware of the child who recognizes that his asthma can be fashioned into an emotional weapon that can be used to manipulate Mum and Dad.

It is a risky business to let asthmatic children get away with behaviour for which their nonasthmatic siblings would be immediately punished. While it is obviously important to appreciate the psychological trauma severe asthma can cause, in most cases it is inadvisable to hold on to the old-fashioned notions that it is the child's 'unhappiness' or 'maladjustment' that is at the root of the ailment. For parents who persist in perpetuating this no-win scenario, and for children who encourage it, a doctor's referral to a psychiatrist or psychologist may be in the best interests of everyone concerned.

Can a child outgrow asthma? There is simply no solid evidence to support the notion that the hormonal changes occurring during puberty will have any effect on your child's asthma condition. To the inevitable question all parents ask, 'Will my child outgrow asthma?' the most honest answer I or any other allergist can give is 'No one knows'. Certainly some children appear to get better as they grow older. But whether *your* child will lose *his* particular symptoms, no one can tell.

One generalization can be made: approximately one-third of all asthmatic children will improve as they grow older; one-third will get worse; one-third will stay the same. Those who improve generally do so by adolescence. Statistics are all well and good when talking to a large audience, of course, but I realize it is a relatively unsatisfactory response in a one-to-one discussion. With all due apologies, it is simply the best that can be done given the present state of our knowledge.

Asthma and your child's heart Though children with severe asthma will often puff and pant, turn red and white in the face and go through such contortions during an attack that parents fear for their very lives it should be stressed that asthma rarely causes damage to the heart. Only under the most unusual circumstances can it cause permanent changes in any organ, including the lungs.

Exercise-induced asthma Physical exertion is often the stimulus that triggers wheezing in asthmatic children. In fact, there are some youngsters who wheeze *only* after periods of strenuous physical exertion, and whose lungs are otherwise normal. This particular type of asthma is called *exercise-induced asthma*, abbreviated as EIA.

Running, football, and rugby are well-known EIA triggers, while cycling, tennis and especially swimming are less likely to bring on attacks. We do know that if exertion takes place in a cool, dry atmosphere, wheezing is more likely to occur than when the weather is warm and humid. In other words, your child may have no problems playing actively during the summer months, but the same activity performed on a windy, wintry day will rapidly produce EIA.

Typically, the child with EIA develops wheezing at the *end* of an exercise period, and the symptoms disappear within thirty to ninety minutes. A small number of children with EIA will also experience a delayed onset of symptoms, beginning four to eight hours after the exercise has ended. This delayed-response pattern tends to produce more severe wheezing than the immediate response and should therefore be carefully monitored. Fortunately the use of specific asthma medications, aerosol beta-adrenergic agents and sodium cromoglycate in particular a few minutes before exertion will usually keep even severe cases of EIA under control. We will discuss these medications shortly.

DIAGNOSING YOUR CHILD'S ASTHMA: HOW IT'S DONE

Wheezing is probably, but not invariably, an indication of asthma. In attempting to diagnose the cause of a wheeze, the first thing you must do is become familiar with asthma's wheeze-causing 'look-alikes', which at first glance sound and look like asthma but stem from entirely different causes. Before taking your wheezing child to a specialist, review the following conditions. They will help you and your doctor home in on the cause of your child's wheezing.

In early infancy, nasal obstruction or congestion can cause a child to produce wheeze-like sounds. These sounds actually originate in the nasal passageways, not in the lungs, and have nothing to do with asthma. In most cases, careful observation by the parents will help differentiate between the two conditions. At times it is difficult without a stethoscope to decide where the wheezing sound originates. A visit to the doctor is recommended if symptoms persist.

In certain very young children there may be an abnormality of the trachea called tracheomalacia. Here the trachea's cartilage rings partially collapse each time a child inhales, creating in the process a wheezing-type sound. Ordinarily, as the child grows older the cartilage rings become stiffer, and the condition corrects itself.

Less common are the so-called webs, rings or slings which exert pressure on the trachea and major bronchi and are formed from anatomical abnormalities of the major blood vessels near the heart. These rings occasionally become so prominent that they partially block the trachea or the oesophagus, producing asthma-like symptoms. This condition requires surgical correction.

Between the ages of one and three, random objects inadvertently swallowed often prove to be the true cause behind respiratory symptoms, especially if wheezing sounds are localized to only one side of the chest. Small, easily swallowable items such as rings, coins, blades of grass, small toys and pebbles are fished out of children every day of the year, and all can produce bronchospasm. The sudden onset of respiratory distress with wheezing should be a signal to get your child to a doctor or casualty department.

Childhood infections such as croup, bronchitis and pneumonia may induce wheezing symptoms parents mistakenly identify as asthma. The same is true with bronchiolitis, a viral respiratory disorder that involves the smaller parts of the breathing tubes and generally strikes infants. Some children who have recurring attacks of bronchiolitis are actually demonstrating the first stage of a genuine asthmatic condition. This pattern tends to be especially true if there is a positive history of asthma or allergy in the family. Your doctor will fill you in on the details. If your child has any respiratory symptoms such as persistent cough, wheeze or shortness of breath, discuss the situation with him.

In addition to the preceding conditions there are a number of other situations in which asthma–like symptoms may be present. These include: anatomic abnormalities of the trachea and bronchial tubes, the rare presence of a cyst or tumour within the respiratory tract, and such medical conditions as cystic fibrosis or tuberculosis. Exposure to toxic chemicals and air pollutants can certainly cause respiratory distress with shortness of breath and wheezing. In order to diagnose most of these conditions a doctor will have to examine your child.

Once you have reason to believe that your child suffers from asthma, the single most important service you can render an allergist is to prepare a thoughtful, complete medical history and to present it at the first visit. Briefly speaking, the most important points to cover include:

when your child's symptoms began

frequency of the child's attacks

particular situations that trigger episodes

medical measures that have been taken in the past

types of medication used

the child's typical level of activities

The more information you supply the specialist at the time of the initial visit, the more specific will be the diagnosis and recommendations. For more details on preparing a child's personal medical history, see the checklist on page 29.

SPECIFIC DIAGNOSTIC TESTS FOR ASTHMA

After examining your child and checking her medical history, the doctor may wish to run several diagnostic tests to determine if asthma is the correct diagnosis. Though the majority of tests used for this purpose have been described on pages 36–47, let's review the common ones and add a few that have not yet been mentioned.

X-ray If there has been a significant increase in a child's respiratory symptoms, if there has been an obvious change in their pattern and frequency, if the child has suffered from breathing problems for a prolonged period of time, and if no chest X-rays have been taken to date, X-ray studies will probably be ordered. They are not a standard procedure, however, and will be called for only when the above conditions prevail.

ECG (Electrocardiogram) Usually an ECG is requested only when there is a history of heart problems or when the physical examination turns up evidence of possible cardiac trouble, such as a heart murmur. If neither of these conditions is present, I would advise that you inquire directly why the ECG has been ordered. Presumably your doctor has specific reasons, but you as a parent are entitled to know about them. The test itself is neither painful nor harmful and may provide the doctor with important data. If a child has suffered from extremely severe asthma and has been repeatedly hospitalized for this condition, the doctor will attempt to get as much information as possible concerning the child's cardiovascular and respiratory systems; then an ECG will probably be ordered.

Allergy tests These include the direct and indirect skin tests discussed at length on pages 41–4. If any of these tests is positive, it does not necessarily mean that the allergen triggering the response is causing asthma, only that it is now a strong possible suspect. After the test results are obtained, the doctor must by means of observation, analysis of the personal medical history, and a synthesis of all that is known concerning the child's condition decide whether a clinical relationship really does exist between asthma and the positive test results.

Blood tests Several may be ordered. These include the FBC or full blood count (see page 36) and the IgE level determination test (see page 37). Another, the quantitative immunoglobulins test (see page 37), is requested mainly for patients demonstrating a pattern of frequent severe bacterial infections. If, in fact, abnormally low levels of certain protective antibodies are found in the bloodstream, patients may require special treatment against such infections.

Sputum test Microscopic studies of sputum or mucus secretions coughed up from the lungs during an attack are rarely done on a routine basis in the case of asthma. It is often difficult to get an adequate specimen from younger children (just ask a two-year-old to cough and spit up on demand), and the result often has little practical application.

Bronchial inhalation challenge tests An allergen believed to be the cause of a child's asthma is inhaled directly in aerosol form, and the patient is observed to see if any signs of an allergic response develop. (Sometimes metacholine or histamine is used in place of specific allergens; both of these trigger wheezing attacks in susceptible subjects but leave nonasthmatics unaffected.) The metacholine and histamine challenge can be used as a differential test to decide if a patient really is asthmatic. Inhalation challenge tests are done in a hospital or consulting room with a doctor in constant attendance so that when and if severe wheezing develops, the appropriate medicine can be quickly administered. If a child reacts to a specific allergen during the test with changes in pulmonary function or with obvious clinical asthma symptoms, then the diagnosis of allergic asthma is confirmed.

Challenge tests are done infrequently, usually only in research establishments, and only when the diagnosis is a difficult one. The test has built-in hazards: provoking an asthmatic attack always creates the possibility of severe symptoms developing, though with proper precautions this procedure can be of great help and provide information essential for the management of the child's condition. If your child is scheduled to take such a test, it is in her best interest to describe beforehand how and where the procedure will be done and that she will not have to remain in the hospital after the test is completed.

Pulmonary function study As soon as a child is old enough to co-operate fully with a doctor – usually around the age of five or six – pulmonary function studies will be ordered (see page 45). Younger children can sometimes be tested with a simple device called a peak flow meter. There is good evidence to suggest that any child with chronic asthma symptoms should be monitored at home with daily peak flow meter determinations. These tests are done with a variety of mechanical devices, both large and small. They are designed to measure the abnormalities typically found in the lungs of a child with chronic asthma and to determine how well the child's lungs are actually working. By and large, this test is quick and painless. The child breathes into a mechanical device and the strength and quality of each breath is recorded, measured and then evaluated by the allergist. Most children with asthma will demonstrate some degree of functional abnormality during these studies, even when no signs of breathing difficulty are evident.

Arterial blood gas determination In severely asthmatic patients, especially those who have experienced long-term, persistent wheezing, the oxygen level in the bloodstream becomes significant: a sizeable decrease in this level, or an increase in the CO_2 (carbon dioxide) level of the blood may warn of impending respiratory failure. When either of these dangerous conditions is noted, very aggressive treatment will be called for including the administration of oxygen and intravenous fluids and the use of bronchodilators and cortisone. Arterial blood gas studies are almost always performed in a hospital setting.

TREATING YOUR CHILD'S ASTHMA

ENVIRONMENTAL CONTROL

The first and perhaps easiest way to treat an asthmatic child is simply to remove the child from the source of the symptoms. If this manoeuvre is impossible, then the child's environment can be manipulated in such a way that exposure to particular allergens will be minimized. If you avoid exposure, you can avoid symptoms.

If, for example, it is known that contact with an animal or a certain food triggers symptoms, everyone involved should realize that the child must be kept away from these allergens.

Simple. But this fact is not as obvious to some as logic might dictate. In my medical practice I am constantly asked by the parents of animal-sensitive children for permission to bring a pet into the home. Despite the child's known susceptibilities to animal dander and despite an observable one-to-one relationship between contact with the allergen and an allergic response, some parents continue to believe that the child will somehow muddle through it all or that the allergy will magically disappear on its own.

But it usually doesn't. In fact, it should be obvious to parents that if a specific substance or circumstance triggered an allergic problem yesterday, then this agent will most likely do the same thing today, perhaps with even greater severity. Until you know for sure that a child has got over his sensitivity to a particular allergen, keep that particular allergen and that particular child very far apart.

CHECKLIST OF POTENTIAL ALLERGENS FOR ASTHMATIC CHILDREN TO AVOID

What allergenic agents trigger asthma in children? What can be done to minimize or neutralize their effects? Here is a representative checklist:

Certain animals Dogs, cats, birds and rabbits in particular are primary causes of allergic asthma. Better tolerated are guinea pigs, hamsters, reptiles and all varieties of fish. If hairy, furry or feathered pets must for whatever reason be kept in the home, they should be banished from the child's bedroom, and preferably from his general area of the house. If possible, keep these animals restricted to one section of the home, ideally in those areas most easily cleaned – i.e. rooms free of dander-gathering fabrics, rugs, upholstered furniture and heavy curtains. An even better solution is to keep the pet permanently out of doors.

Feathers These are found primarily in bedding, sleeping bags and stuffed furniture. It is a good policy to keep all allergic asthmatic children away from down and from all types of birds. Feather-sensitive children can usually wear down jerkins or coats, but they will find it difficult to sleep under a down quilt *all night* without experiencing symptoms. In other words, the intensity of the exposure determines if symptoms will or will not develop.

Wool Found in carpets, blankets and in woollen clothing such as shirts, dresses, socks, scarves, etc. I am often asked whether or not an allergic asthmatic child can wear a woollen coat. The answer is usually yes, except children who develop skin rashes from wool.

Dusty environments Shun them. Dust is both an allergen and a just-plain-irritating substance. Exposure to a room full of dust can cause nasal congestion, sneezing and for many children an asthma attack. To help combat irritating inhalants, filtering devices can be used to clean the air of dust, cigarette smoke, pollens and a variety of other allergens. See pages 49–54 for detailed information.

Moulds Household areas such as attics and cellars are predisposed to mould growth and should be avoided. In many cases dampness will cause asthma and so will moulds. The combination of the two can be a disaster.

Controlled humidity During the winter, when heating units make homes arid and hot, it is best to keep the indoor relative humidity between 35 and 45 per cent, even if an electronic humidifier must be installed to do the trick (see page 50).

Heating systems Be aware of the effects of household heating systems. The worst from the viewpoint of an asthmatic child is the forced-air type. The hot billows of bone-dry air that pour out of these units stir up room dust like small cyclones and tend to dry out the mucous membranes of the throat. Steam radiators are something of an improvement, and skirting-board heating is better still. Excellent, though most expensive, is radiant electric heat. Now that I have condemned forced-air heating, however, it should be noted that a forced-air system supplied with a built-in humidifier and an electronic filter is a wonderful set-up for environmentally controlled living. In fact, a system of this kind is probably the very best of all possible heating arrangements in a household with an allergic or asthmatic family member.

Air conditioning In most instances, air conditioning is an aid for allergy and asthma sufferers. The one exception is the case of the child who is especially sensitive to abrupt changes of air temperature and whose breathing becomes suddenly laboured whenever she enters an air-conditioned house on a hot summer day. In such instances air conditioning is obviously more of a liability than an asset and should not be used. Do not make the mistake of thinking that an air conditioner filters the air of all undesirable particles. It doesn't, at least not to any dependable degree. To remove ultrafine particles typical of smoke, pollen, moulds and other minute allergens, special air-filtration systems will almost always be necessary (see page 49).

ASTHMA MEDICATIONS FOR YOUR CHILD: AS COMPLETE A SURVEY AS YOU'LL EVER NEED

First, a word of warning: if your child suffers from bronchial asthma, do not self-medicate him; use only drugs prescribed by a qualified doctor.

This said, we can get to the business of describing the most commonly prescribed asthma medicines. While it may seem to the bewildered parent that there are an endless number of these medications, they are, in fact, rather limited. All the asthma drugs you may have run across through the years are simply varieties and brand names of the same small number of drug families.

BRONCHODILATORS

Theophylline

Theophylline is prescribed under a variety of brand names and has been used to treat bronchial asthma since 1937. Its use is subject to considerable dissension in the medical profession. Paediatricians still seem to like it but adult chest specialists are going off it and the actual number of theophylline and related compounds prescribable has reduced sharply in recent years, although new products are still coming on the market with claims to overcome some of the previous shortcomings.

Slo-Phyllin, Theo-Dur and Phyllocontin are some of the more popular names you may come across. A more definitive list can be found in Table 3.

How does it work? In many ways. Most importantly, it relaxes the smooth muscle surrounding the bronchi or breathing tubes, thereby reducing obstruction of the lungs. It also stimulates the cilia, those millions of tiny hairlike follicles lining the airways which serve to propel mucus up and out of the lungs, keeping the respiratory system clean of excess secretions and cellular debris. Theophylline also stimulates the central nervous system during asthmatic episodes, specifically the respiratory centre. Lastly, there is some evidence that theophylline improves the muscle function of both the diaphragm and various other respiratory muscles, thus strengthening the lungs during an attack. In all, a highly useful and efficacious medication.

In more recent years knowledge of theophylline's chemistry

has increased and its blood levels can be determined. This has gone some way to making it a more acceptable drug, but some doctors still have strong reservations.

Limitations and side effects Theophylline is a highly effective bronchodilator for most children, but not for all. Some simply cannot tolerate it; others have such an erratic metabolism that it becomes almost impossible to regulate dosages. Certain children tolerate the drug quite well in such low doses as perhaps not to be clinically effective.

In general, it can be said that a majority of theophylline's side effects stem from too high a dose, not from the action of the drug itself. You are advised to become familiar with these side effects (as well as those of any other medication your child is taking), and to carefully describe any questionable symptoms to your doctor. The signs and symptoms to watch for with theophylline overdose consist of the following:

Nausea, loss of appetite, vomiting and heartburn.

Rapid heartbeat, palpitations and in a few very rare cases irregular heart rhythms. This in no way means that theophylline causes cardiac problems or that it damages the heart. Symptoms vanish as soon as the medication is stopped.

Headaches, restlessness and insomnia. While it has not been proved, there is also a possibility that some children taking theophylline on a daily schedule may experience a decrease in their ability to concentrate. If this should occur, stopping the drug eliminates the problem.

Hyperactivity. Some children become hyperactive even though the amount of theophylline in their bloodstream is well within the normal treatment range. Such patients are simply unable to tolerate this medicine regardless of the amount administered.

Quite a list. But remember, these symptoms develop only in a small minority of children who are on theophylline. If you are aware of the potential problems, then the medicine can be discontinued or changed at the earliest signs of trouble.

Still, there are youngsters who suffer some side effects of theophylline even when the drug is administered in appropriate dosages. Headaches may occur, as well as heartburn, nausea, hyperactivity. If these reactions continue, it means that your child's body chemistry is simply not compatible with the drug. If the dose is readjusted several times and there is still no improvement, a new medication must be tried. It must, however, be stressed once again that most children, when given a carefully regulated dose of theophylline, can take it for long periods of time without developing adverse reactions of any kind.

Clearance rate Many conditions such as age, weight and diet affect the way a child metabolizes any medication. These conditions will cause the body either to increase the speed at which the medicine is used up or to slow it down. The measurement of how rapidly the body consumes a specific drug is known as the *clearance rate*, and this rate will vary from child to child. As a rule, children metabolize theophylline more quickly than adults and require more of the substance per pound of body weight. Table 1 illustrates how clearance rates work with regard to several critical variables.

What exactly does the clearance rate tell us about the way a child reacts to theophylline and to medications in general? A *decreased* clearance rate means that the drug is remaining in the child's system longer than was expected and that it may be reaching a toxic level in the blood with resultant side effects. An *increased* rate causes the drug to be used up faster than was expected, lowering the amount of drug in the bloodstream so that it fails to produce the anticipated therapeutic effects.

There are, in addition to the conditions listed above, children who by nature are either rapid or slow metabolizers of theophylline. This means that for these children it will be necessary to monitor closely the amount of theophylline in the blood. Ideally, any child who will be taking a theophylline preparation on a long-term basis will require periodic theophylline blood level determinations, but this is not always practicable.

Dosage Naturally, it is the doctor's responsibility to prescribe the appropriate dose of theophylline, but as a parent you must have a general understanding of how the doctor arrives at the theophylline dose for your child.

The dose is decided by two factors, both of which have a strong bearing on the way the child utilizes the drug: age and weight. Table 2 provides a guide to dosage strengths. Use it to determine whether or not your child is receiving medication within the range appropriate for age and weight. If something seems out of the ordinary, do not come to hasty conclusions until you consult your doctor – it must be stressed that the figures in Table 2 are based on averages and are not chiselled in stone. Most likely it will turn out that there is sound method to the doctor's decisions.

Blood tests Ideally, all children who are taking theophylline regularly should have a periodic (every six months) blood test done in order to determine if they are receiving the correct dose of medicine. If a youngster will be on theophylline for only a relatively short time (less than two weeks) and he is doing well on the medication, there is no need for a theophylline level determination.

The main reason for doing this test is to let everyone know if the prescribed dose of theophylline is providing the patient with a therapeutic blood level. The optimal effective level of theophylline in the circulation is between 10 and 20 micrograms per millilitre of blood. Levels above this range are frequently associated with signs and symptoms of theophylline toxicity. When the circulating level is under 10 micrograms per millilitre, the bronchodilating effect of theophylline is definitely decreased, though I have had patients who are clinically well with theophylline levels of less than 10 micrograms.

Table 1 Theopylline Blood Levels

Factors that can increase circulating levels of theophylline

High-carbohydrate diet	Heart failure
Drugs: Cimetidine (Tagamet)	Kidney failure
Clindamycin	Liver failure
Erythromycin estolate	Viral infections
Troleandomycin (TAD)	Pulmonary oedema

Factors that can decrease circulating levels of theophylline

High-protein diet   Charcoal-grilled foods   Smoking tobacco or marijuana

Young children (under five) rapidly metabolize theophylline. They therefore require higher doses based on their weight than older children or adolescents.

Table 2 Theophylline Dose Recommendations

Age or predisposing condition	Milligrams of theophylline per kilogram of body weight* per twenty-four-hour period
Children	
12 months–9 years	18–20
9–16 years Young adult smokers	16
Adults	
Healthy, nonsmoking	10
Over 50 with heart condition	6
Children or Adults	
Congestive heart failure	5
Liver disease	2.4

NOTE: It is always safer to begin treatment with a dose approximately two-thirds of the recommended amount and gradually increase the dose to the recommended level. For any patient who will be maintained on a constant regimen of theophylline, it is important to check the theophylline blood level periodically.

*The proper dose of theophylline should be based on a person's *ideal* or *lean* body weight.

How do these tests work? Most likely your doctor will want to check the drug's peak level first. This test is performed when the maximum amount of theophylline is circulating in the system: one to two hours after a short-acting form of the drug has been administered; four to five hours after a long-acting or sustained-release form is used. A small amount of blood is taken from a vein or a finger stick to be analysed.

If there are major problems with regulating the theophylline dose, it may also be necessary to check the trough, or lowest blood level. This level is reached just before the effects of the drug are wearing off, when the patient is ready for a new dose (this can be anywhere from six to eight or even twelve hours after the medicine has been administered). It is unusual to get a trough level determination, and in practice it is usually necessary to check only the peak level.

The concept of therapeutic drug monitoring – checking the amount of medicine circulating in the bloodstream – is an accepted practice in all fields of medicine, but as with any new medical procedure, costs are high and widespread availability of the tests is still limited.

These tests are not uncommon in hospital practice but GPs tend more to rely on their clinical judgement.

There has been a decline in the number of theophylline preparations because the short-acting forms gave a high incidence of side effects, but since sustained-release forms have become available their use has been increased. With the many varieties available there is the problem of knowing which preparation is best for a particular case. This problem can be somewhat simplified by adding a few facts to what you already know about theophylline.

Until ten years ago, theophylline was prepared commercially in combination with a variety of other drugs. For many asthmatic patients these combination preparations were quite effective, but for others, especially children, they were poorly tolerated and side effects abounded. Also, if patients needed an increased dose of theophylline it was necessary to take elevated amounts of all the other drugs as well, as they came together in fixed drug combinations. Today we know that fixed drug combinations are certainly not appropriate preparations for treating childhood asthma symptoms. In those situations when a patient on theophylline requires additional medication to control her asthma, a second bronchodilator preparation can be added as a supplement. This is a benefit, of course, for when drugs are prescribed individually rather than in fixed combinations the doctor maintains control over the appropriate dose of each, gaining the best results while minimizing side effects.

Theophylline comes in two basic forms: short-acting and long-acting or sustained-release. The short-acting forms are available in liquid, tablets, chewable tablets or capsules. They are usually taken once every six hours and reach a peak level in the bloodstream within one to two hours.

The long-acting or sustained-release preparations are available as tablets, capsules, and the so-called sprinkle forms. Sprinkles are capsules filled with hundreds of tiny beads that are shaken directly on to foods such as apple sauce and are then swallowed along with the food. Do not let the child chew these granules. They taste terrible and chewing will destroy their long-acting properties.

Although for an acute wheezing attack one of the short-acting forms of theophyllines would be the most appropriate of this type of drug, it is more likely that one of the beta-adrenergic agents will be used. Theophylline in its sustained-release form is often used at night as a single dose to control nocturnal wheezing or is administered every twelve hours to control the more chronic forms of asthma. Because of its twelve-hourly action there is the advantage of not having to wake children at night or to interrupt their studies at school to give the medicines.

Stick as closely as possible to a regular schedule for the administration of theophylline. Dosage times should become as familiar and habitual to your child's daily living rhythms as lunchtime or bedtime. If for whatever reason a child does miss her dose, do *not* make it up by giving a double dose next time. The treatment range and the toxic range of theophylline are rather close, and too much given at one time can easily cause side effects.

Theophylline is such a bitter-tasting chemical that drug manufacturers have found it impossible to produce a truly palatable liquid form. Children usually down the pills and the capsules and especially the sprinkles without a major struggle, but even adults cannot tolerate the liquid. This is especially problematic in the case of very young children who have difficulty swallowing pills and who must take the liquid form or none at all. In such cases, remember that the more concentrated the liquid, the less medicine your child must swallow (strengths are listed on the bottle). You might also try making the portion more acceptable by mixing it with a strong sweetener. Parents have reported some measure of success with standard seductions such as maple syrup.

Table 3 gives a list of the most commonly used forms of theophylline and the related xanthine drugs aminophylline and choline theophyllinate.

Other potential dangers Though theophylline is ordinarily a safe drug, as with all medications, misuse can cause trouble and even danger. The most important thing for parents to realize in this regard is that *under no circumstances should they attempt to medicate a child with theophylline* without medical guidance. Occasionally parents with more than one asthmatic child will have a surplus of the drug on hand and they will randomly give Johnny's medication to Suzie during an attack. THIS IS A SERIOUS MISTAKE. The precise theophylline dose, as we have seen, is a critical factor in treatment, not only to ensure the best clinical response but to avoid potentially dangerous side effects.

BETA-ADRENERGIC AGENTS (OR DRUGS)

Beta-adrenergic agents are a group of drugs chemically related to adrenaline which, like theophylline, belong to the bronchodilator drug family. During the past two decades, chemists and clinical pharmacologists have produced a constant stream of these preparations, so that today the beta-adrenergic class of bronchodilators represent the fastest-growing area of asthma pharmacotherapy.

Side effects Skeletal-muscle tremor is perhaps the most frequent side-effect of these drugs. In a child a common indication of this side effect is an obvious worsening of penmanship, sometimes clearly visible trembling of the hands. Teachers will complain that a child who has been an attentive pupil now can't seem to sit still. Fortunately most children will tolerate this symptom, and within five to seven days the shakiness will disappear. This problem

Table 3 Commonly Prescribed Theophylline Preparations

Brand name	Strength	Colour	Usual dosage (interval in hours)	Scored tablets (availability)
Liquids				
Biophylline	125mg/5ml	Clear	6–8	
Nuflin liquid	60mg/5ml	Brown		
Related Drugs				
Phyllocontin Paediatric tablets (Aminophylline)	100mg	Pale orange	12	No
Choledyl (Choline theophyllinate)	100mg	Pink	6–8	No
Choledyl	200mg	Yellow	6–8	No
Choledyl syrup	62.5mg/5ml			
Short-acting tablets				
Nuelin	125mg	White	6–8	Yes
Long-acting tablets				
Nuelin SA	175mg	White	12	No
Nuelin SA-250	250mg	White	12	Yes
Theo-Dur	200mg	Off-white mottled oval	12	Yes
Uniphyllin Paediatric continus	200mg	White	24	Yes
Long-acting capsules				
Slo-Phyllin	60mg	White/clear white pellets	12	No
Slo-Phyllin	125mg	Brown/clear white pellets	12	No
Slo-Phyllin	250mg	Blue/clear blue & white pellets	12	No

appears in only 10 to 25 per cent of children who are started on this class of bronchodilators.

Other less frequent complaints include rapid heartbeat (tachycardia) and bouts of insomnia. Parents occasionally report that their child has become extremely hyperactive while being treated, and occasionally I hear of a usually well-behaved child suddenly going haywire when using these medicines. In such cases the medication must of course be adjusted or discontinued.

What follows is a discussion of the most commonly used preparations.

Adrenaline

Twenty years ago adrenaline was the mainstay of the management of acute asthma. It had to be given by injection with the needle point just under the skin and the injection given very slowly. The rule was 'a minim a minute' (a minim being approximately 1/17 of 1 ml) to a patient who had not had adrenaline before, but patients who were used to the drug built up a considerable tolerance and could take it faster. The drug was often self-administered and was very effective if not overused. However, there were considerable dangers especially if, by accident, the drug was injected into a blood vessel; this could prove fatal. It could produce a violent jittering or shaky feeling: we all know the expression 'the adrenaline flowing' – well, that was literally what it was like. In its day it was indispensable but now it has been superseded by more modern drugs and is very rarely used in this country.

Ephedrine

The other mainstay of treatment was the ephedrine tablet. It was given either alone or in a number of combinations with other drugs. It, too, has had its day and has been overtaken by more modern medicaments, and you are unlikely to come across it.

Isoprenaline

This drug stimulates both the heart and lungs, sometimes to such a degree that the rapid heartbeat becomes a distressing side effect.

It is most effective when used as an aerosol. Though a standby for years as a proven asthma medication, isoprenaline has a comparatively short duration of action when measured against the newer, more effective drugs. It is now outdated and considered less suitable and safe than the beta-adrenergic agents.

Orciprenaline

This is known as a partially selective beta-agonist; in other words it favours bronchodilation while still stimulating the heart to some extent. It is marketed under the name of Alupent. It comes in the form of tablets, syrup, and MDI and an injection. It has been used effectively and safely with very young children.

Salbutamol

Probably the most widely prescribed asthma drug today is salbutamol, chiefly known under its trade name of Ventolin but also marketed under a number of other names such as Asmaven, Cobutalin, and Salbulin. Salbutamol comes in a variety of different forms: 2 mg and 4 mg tablets, a long-lasting 8 mg tablet called a Spandet, in a syrup form 2 mg/5 ml, and as an injection. All these, of course, except the injection, are taken by mouth, and they act by being absorbed into the bloodstream, by which they are carried to the lungs, where they have the effect of dilating the breathing tubes, as the name bronchodilator implies. However, if the drug is inhaled it is carried directly to its target area and a much smaller quantity is needed, since it does not have to be widely dispersed through the bloodstream to have its effect. There are three ways in which bronchodilator drugs can be inhaled:

> *As an inhaler or MDI (metered dose inhaler)*
> This is a small hand-held pump which delivers a metered dose of aerosol when the top is pushed in. The dose per actuation of the pump is 100 mg (compare this with the dose by the oral route; it is 1/20 of the smallest tablet or one teaspoonful of the syrup).
>
> Although the pumps are simple in construction and actuation, their proper use must be taught to ensure that the

patient is using them correctly. Dummy MDIs are available which do not deliver a dose of salbutamol but in other respects are identical. These can be used in the surgery when the correct technique is being taught.

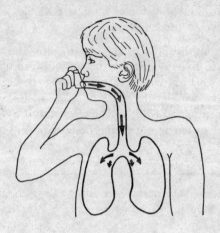

Figure 3 How to use a metered dose inhaler

The spray released when you discharge a gas-propelled, hand-held metered dose inhaler leaves the mouthpiece at approximately sixty to seventy miles per hour. In other words, the medicine doesn't take very long to reach its destination, and if your child does not accurately synchronize her inhalation with the spray, very little of the medicine will ever reach her lungs. When you visit the doctor, ask for specific directions on how to use this device. Go over these directions several times.

For handy reference, here are the fundamentals of MDI use:

1. Shake the inhaler for several seconds before using. The part that holds the medicine, the canister, must be held upright and positioned *above* the mouthpiece during use.

2. It is best to use the inhaler while standing up.

3. Open your mouth, place the nozzle of the inhaler in your mouth and close your lips around it. As you begin to breathe in, squeeze the canister and continue to inhale the spray for as long as possible, usually about two to three seconds.

4. Close your mouth, hold your breath, and count silently to five.

5. When you finally exhale, do so slowly, as if breathing out through a straw.

   Wait five to ten minutes, then repeat steps 3, 4 and 5.

Salbutamol is a very safe drug. It starts to work very quickly, within two to five minutes, and the therapeutic effect can last from four to six hours in most patients. It produces side effects of muscle trembling and a feeling of shakiness well below a dose that is toxic. Nevertheless, a maximum dose of 1–2 puffs three to four times per day is put on the use of an MDIs. This is because if it is not producing the required bronchodilator effect within this dose, there is something wrong. Frequently it is just poor use technique. Some children get the hang of inhaling and actuating the pump correctly without any difficulty, probably more easily than adults! Some never seem to master it, and telltale puffs at the corners of the mouth show that a lot of the aerosol is escaping. Re-educating them in MDI technique solves some of the problems, or change to, or addition of, another form of medication may be required.

As a Rotacap

This is a capsule containing salbutamol in powder form. It is inserted into a small hand-held device called a Rotahaler, where a simple twisting action breaks open the capsule releasing the powder. The device is placed in the mouth and a sharp intake of breath sucks the powder into the lungs. Some patients find this easier than using the aerosol properly; on the other hand, some do not like the sensation of powder being inhaled into the lungs; but even if there is initial dislike, this is usually overcome with perseverance. The Rotacap/Rotahaler method is possibly marginally more effective than the aerosol; a larger portion of the drug seems to get into the lungs.

The Rotahaler is slightly less convenient to use than the aerosol. Whereas the aerosol can be used quickly with one hand, the other method involves taking a capsule out of a box, inserting it into the device and twisting it, using both hands, before inhalation. This does not sound much, but it is less easy to do without other people noticing and some patients are embarrassed to be seen to need medication. In view of these minor difficulties some patients have a Rotahaler at home which can be used morning and evening and an aerosol which can be slipped in the pocket and used quickly and unobtrusively away from home and in company.

Warning: When *any* MDI is used, be attentive to the way the child handles it and be on the lookout for abuse. If a medicine works well, it is only human nature for parents to haul it out every time their child's condition takes a turn for the worse, even a small turn. In the hands of a youngster who has no real sense of the potential toxicity of a drug, the temptation to use it at will is twice as great, and surreptitious overuse can become a dangerous habit. Many children under twelve are not mature enough to handle the responsibility which the self-administration of any strong medicine requires, and it is suggested that parents *never* give a child *carte blanche* with an inhaler or, for that matter, with a potent medicine of any kind.

As a help in this direction, note that most hand-held aerosolized nebulizers contain approximately 200 sprays. So make it a habit to record the date on which the canister is first put into use, then make a note of the day on which it becomes empty. In this way you will be able to monitor how many sprays per day are being taken. If the number is larger than ten (that is, if the medicine is used up within twenty days or less) a serious discussion should take place between the patient, parents and doctor.

By nebulizer
This will be discussed later (page 137).

OTHER BETA-ADRENERGIC AGENTS

Terbutaline

This drug is used under the brand name of Bricanyl. There is a similar range to salbutamol of different presentations of the drug, excluding the Rotahaler delivery system. It is very useful in having a longer duration of action than salbutamol.

One of the problems with the MDI system is that of poor technique; also the particles leave the nozzle of the MDI at a high speed, which leads to the great majority of the drug sticking to the back of the throat and then being swallowed. Only about 10 per cent of the aerosol leaving the MDI actually gets to the respiratory tract. If the aerosol is squirted into a chamber the particles are slowed down, then the aerosol mist can be inhaled from the chamber more effectively. The makers of Bricanyl have made use of this in two ways:

> There is a form of MDI which incorporates a folding chamber called a spacer which is pulled out in front of the nozzle.

> They also supply a larger plastic chamber called a Nebuhaler, which looks like a clear plastic cocktail shaker. It fits on to the front of the standard MDI and is rather bulky and cumbersome. These extension chambers can be used only with the Bricanyl MDI. They both ensure that a larger portion of the aerosol is inhaled into the lungs.

Fenoterol (Berctec), pirbuterol (Exirel), reproterol (Bronchodil) are all drugs of this class which are delivered by MDIs. Rimiterol (Pulmadil) is delivered both by an MDI and by a breath–actuated inhaler. (See Figure 4.)

The third class of bronchodilator are the anti–cholinergic

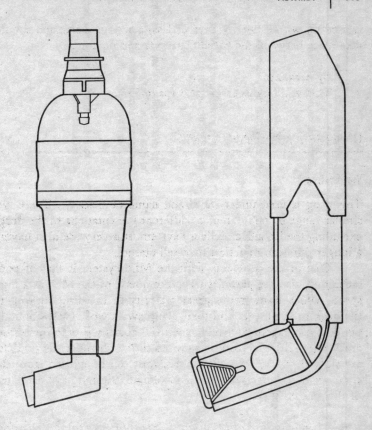

Figure 4

agents. At present the only one in routine use is ipratropium bromide (Atrovent). It works in a completely different pharmacological fashion to the beta-adrenergic agents and so can be used to supplement them. It is given by an MDI; initially the amount per dose was too small and so a double-strength Atrovent Forte has been introduced. There is also a combined MDI which gives ipratropium bromide with the beta-adrenergic agent fenoterol under the brand name Duovent. Ipratropium bromide can also be given by nebulizer. Although the makers recommend its use only to those over the age of three, it has been used safely in very young children. The receptors that mediate the use of the beta-adrenergic

Table 4 Beta-adrenergic Bronchodilators

Generic name	Brand name	How administered	Dosage	Comments & side effects
Adrenaline		By injection	Slowly as single dose	Jitteriness, nausea, rapid heartbeat.
Isoprenaline	Aleudrin	Tablet (dissolved under tongue)	1–3/day	As above, both rarely used now.
	Iso Autohaler	MDI	1–3 puffs repeated after 30 minutes. Maximum 24 puffs in 24 hrs	
Ephedrine	Medihaler Iso	MDI Tablet Elixir	3 times daily	Similar to adrenaline but less effect on heart. Difficulty in passing urine.
Orciprenaline	Alupent	Tablet Syrup MDI Injection	3–4 times daily " " Maximum 12 puffs in 24 hrs. May be repeated after 30 minutes	Side effects similar to those of adrenaline or isoprenaline. Shakiness due to muscle tremor most annoying side effect. Minimized by giving orally.
Salbutamol	Ventolin	Tablet Syrup Long-acting tablets MDI Rotacap/Rotahaler Nebulizer Injection	3–4 times a day " " " 12 hourly 1–2 puffs 3–4 times a day 3–4 times a day As directed by doctor Single dose or may be repeated	Fewer side effects than other beta agents but muscle tremor can occur.
	Salbulin	Tablet MDI	3–4 times a day. 1–2 puffs 3–4 times a day	

Terbutaline	Bricanyl	Tablet Syrup Long-acting tablet MDI Nebulizer solution Injection	8–12 hourly " " 12 hourly 1–2 puffs as required up to 8 in 24 hrs As directed by doctor Single dose or may be repeated	Side effects as above. Longer duration of action than salbutamol.
Fenoterol	Berotec	MDI Nebulizer	Up to 2 puffs in 4 hrs As directed by doctor	As above.
Pirbuterol	Exirel	Capsule Syrup MDI	3–4 times a day " " " 1–2 puffs as required up to 12 puffs in 24 hrs	As above.
Reproterol	Bronchodil	Tablet Elixir MDI Nebulizer solution	3 times daily " " Up to 2 puffs 3 times daily As directed by doctor	As above.
Rimiterol	Pulmodil Pulmodil Auto	MDI Breath-actuated MDI	1–3 doses repeated after 30 minutes. Maximum 24 doses in 24 hours	Rapid action.

agents are not fully active in the first year of life, whereas ipratropium bromide is effective in young children.

A small extension chamber is available for use with Duovent.

The role of beta-adrenergic agents Bronchodilator drugs have made great advances in recent years, but they still only control symptoms and cannot cure the disease. For many years after their introduction it was found that the asthma death rate did not drop as expected and it was suspected that the drugs were dangerous. Now the thinking is that too much reliance was placed on their use and that patients continued to increase the dose beyond the useful range, whereas they should have consulted their doctor and had their medication changed.

Beta-adrenergic aerosols are especially effective in blocking the development of exercise-induced asthma.

Aerosolized beta-adrenergic preparations can be taken *in advance* when parents know that their child is entering an allergy-sensitive environment – for example, when visiting someone who owns animals or when travelling from the city to the country during pollen season. As a case in point, if Tim is allergic to Aunt Mary's cat and if there is a family function being held at her home, the MDI can be used ten minutes before the party begins. Tim then has a good chance of passing a pleasant afternoon visiting his relatives rather than spending his day outside the house having an asthma attack.

Preventive medication

Sodium cromoglycate The bronchodilator medicines we have discussed so far are all used to control asthma symptoms once they begin. Sodium cromoglycate (Intal), on the other hand, has a prophylactic action. This means it can block allergic reactions *before* they begin; it can also decrease to some extent the hyper-irritability of the bronchial tree. In my opinion, for most patients who require chronic medication, sodium cromoglycate (Intal) should be considered along with theophylline as a first-line treatment for asthma.

As with any medication, Intal will not be effective for all

patients. Sticking to a regular dosing schedule will definitely increase the chances that Intal will control your child's asthma.

How does it work? As mentioned earlier, asthmatic children have hyper-reactivity of the bronchial airways as a basic physiological abnormality. Sodium cromoglycate, taken on a regular basis (four times a day), has the potential to diminish this increased responsiveness. It also blocks the release from the mast cells of histamine and other asthma-causing substances.

An example of this drug in action concerns Jason, whose best friend happened to own a large, friendly calico cat. Whenever Jason walked into his friend's house, he felt entirely normal. Within ten minutes he began to cough and wheeze, and a few minutes after that he was in the midst of a full-fledged asthmatic attack. When it was determined that the animal was causing the trouble, Jason's doctor prescribed Intal and told Jason to take the drug immediately before entering cat territory. Now Jason plays regularly at his friend's house for two to three hours at a time without any discomfort – but only when he remembers to take his medicine beforehand.

When is Intal prescribed? An increasing number of allergists today consider Intal, along with theophylline and the beta-adrenergic agents, to be a first-line drug, which means that many children do well on it alone and require no further medication. As stated, however, Intal is prophylactic: it must be taken *before* an asthma attack has started, when the lung passageways are free of obstruction. Once bronchospasms begin and the child is actively wheezing, Intal is largely ineffective.

Because it is a prophylactic drug and must be taken three to four times a day in order to be effective, Intal should be prescribed only for children who suffer from chronic asthma and require medication on an ongoing basis. Except in certain specific situations (mentioned below where exercise-induced asthma is discussed), it is by no means a one-time medicine.

Intal must sometimes be taken for several weeks before its full effectiveness becomes apparent. A fair trial is always in order: the child should take one capsule by Spinhaler or two puffs with the MDI four times a day for four to six weeks. If, and only if, there is no clinical improvement whatsoever at the end of this period you can assume that Intal is not effective for your child.

Intal is particularly effective in blocking the type of asthma that results from strenuous physical exertion, known as EIA. Taking one capsule by Spinhaler or two puffs of the MDI twenty minutes before break, gym class or general playtime is an effective way to keep an active child symptom free. When administered immediately before exposure to an allergen such as animal dander, Intal can also suppress an allergic response.

How is the drug administered? Sodium cromoglycate is currently available in three dosage forms: in a metered-dose inhaler, as a powder (in a capsule) and as a solution (in a glass ampoule). The powder is inhaled from a small hand-held device called a Spinhaler. For younger patients who cannot use the Spinhaler, the sodium cromoglycate solution is used with a small compressed air pump. The air pump converts the solution to an aerosol mist that the patient inhales through a face mask.

The mechanics of the Spinhaler operation are as follows:

The sodium cromoglycate (Intal) capsule is placed in the Spinhaler.

The capsule is punctured by sliding the barrel of the Spinhaler down and up.

The child places the Spinhaler in his mouth and inhales deeply. It may take two to six deep breaths to empty the powder from the capsule.

To help young children to achieve a strong sucking action to empty the capsule properly, the makers of Intal have produced a whistle which is attached to the end of the Spinhaler so that the more strongly the child sucks, the louder the whistle sounds. Although it may be very effective in getting the child to use the Spinhaler correctly, the parents may not always thank you as they have to put up with a piercing shriek every time the child uses his Spinhaler!

Side effects Extended studies of sodium cromoglycate show a very low incidence of harmful side effects, and those which do occur are generally quite mild. The most common symptoms are coughing, a transient wheeze, or a slight sore throat.

The starting dose is one capsule four times a day. This schedule is continued for one month. Those patients who have a good response may be continued on as little as two capsules a day. If your child should wheeze or cough after inhaling Intal, this reaction can almost always be blocked by pre-treatment with an aerosolized beta-adrenergic bronchodilator. The bronchodilator MDI dose inhaler should be used five minutes before taking Intal. Generally speaking, sodium cromoglycate is one of the safest drugs on the asthma and allergy market today.

There is, however, one area in which problems may arise. It is not from the drug itself, ironically, but from the patient, the patient's family and the doctor. If he fails to stress the importance of complying with instructions for the use of sodium cromoglycate and does not demonstrate the proper handling of the Spinhaler, the patient is unlikely to make the proper use of the medicine. Why?

The major problem associated with the successful long-term administration of any medication is compliance. Most people just don't like taking medicine, and that is doubly true if you don't feel ill! If Intal is working effectively, your child will have few or no asthma symptoms. It is at this time that you as a parent must be most diligent in making sure that the medicine is taken regularly.

The other concern shared by parents and doctors regarding the use of chronic medication relates to the possible harmful side effects caused by the specific drug. On this point let me reassure you that sodium cromoglycate is one of the safest medications I have prescribed in the past twenty years. Studies carried out world-wide confirm my personal observations.

If this medicine is prescribed for your child, I urge you to give it a fair trial before making a decision about its effectiveness.

Corticosteroids

General comments The many steroid preparations available today are all derived from cortisone, a natural hormone producing by the adrenal glands, those cap-shaped, adrenaline-producing organs located above the kidneys. Steroids have been used for the treatment of severe asthma and other allergic conditions for the past twenty years, and they have undoubtedly saved the lives of many, many children, but they are a double-edged sword. On the one hand, steroids have the ability to relieve a great deal of suffering; on the other, they can cause much misery. The responsibility for steering you through these potentially dangerous waters falls squarely on the doctor's shoulders.

What are these dangers? The list of potential side effects caused by cortisone reads like a pathology textbook. They range from trifles such as increased appetite to extremely serious conditions such as limitation of physical growth, increased incidence of fractured bones, cataracts and ulcer formation.

At this point you may be making a vow never to let your child be treated with corticosteroids of any kind – ever. On the basis of what has been said, I can hardly blame you, but I hope that when you read the pages that follow you will be reassured that if cortisone is prescribed in an appropriate dose and for a short period of time, the chances of serious side effects are extremely small. Indeed, in the overall scheme of asthma therapy, it is absolutely necessary for you to understand when steroids should and should not be used, and to place them in their deserved perspective:

> Cortisone and its derivatives should *not* be the first medicine given for an acute asthma attack. When first administered they can take as long as four to eight hours to work, and this is simply too long.

> Theophylline and the beta-adrenergic bronchodilators should be the first drugs to be used for an acute asthmatic attack. Only if these medications fail to control symptoms adequately should cortisone be considered.

> If a decision has been made to use a cortisone preparation, then it should be administered in the proper dosage and for the shortest period of time needed to do its job, usually less than ten to fourteen days.

If cortisone is to be used for five days or less, there is
no reason to taper the dose: i.e., reduce it from five
pills a day to four, then to three, etc. For example, a
dose of four pills a day can be given for five straight
days and then abruptly discontinued.

The dose *should* be tapered if cortisone is to be given
for more than a week.

Of the many cortisone derivative preparations commercially available I prefer to use an intermediate-acting
form such as prednisone or methyl-prednisolone. These
agents have had a somewhat lower incidence of harmful
side effects than the longer-acting forms of cortisone
such as dexamethasone and betamethasone.

How do they work? Cortisone works in the following ways to help
control asthma:

Because of its ability to reduce inflammation (anti-inflammatory property), it decreases the irritation and mucous congestion in the bronchial tubes.

The lungs respond better to the bronchodilator drugs the
patient is taking.

There is some evidence, but no conclusive proof, that steroids
relax the bronchial smooth muscle spasms that are a major
problem for all children with asthma.

Remember that the clinical effects of cortisone are not apparent
until two to eight hours after the medicine has been taken.

How are corticosteroids administered? Cortisone and its derivatives
may be administered in tablet form, as a liquid, by injection or
intravenously.

Most commonly steroids are administered orally, either as a
liquid or tablet. Intravenous methods are generally limited to
hospital, while injections are rarely necessary and are used only
when the doctor suspects that the patient is not taking the medicine

as prescribed. Table 5 (on page 124) provides the names of the most commonly used oral forms.

Side effects While a child is taking cortisone, parents should be certain that the doctor makes constant efforts to decrease both the dose and the length of time the drug is given. As there is a direct relationship between dose, duration of treatment, and the development of side effects, the possibility of overuse must be meticulously guarded against by everyone involved.

This is an extremely critical point to understand. Cortisone rarely causes problems when treatment is limited to a five- to ten-day course. When given for more than two weeks, side effects will probably begin, albeit lesser ones such as increased appetite or weight gain. If daily treatment continues for a month or more, potentially serious adverse effects can and do often occur. These may include:

a decrease in the function of the adrenal glands

a slowing of the child's growth rate. (If given for long enough in a high enough dose, steroids can induce premature closure of the growth centres in the bones, stopping the child's physical growth *entirely*.)

a decrease in resistance to infection

changes in the skin, with a tendency to the development of acne, stretch marks and excess body hair

adverse effects on the contours of the child's face, producing what is called a 'moon facies' – an exaggerat-edly rounded or 'moon face'

headaches, insomnia and dizziness

stomach and intestinal problems, with the possibility of stomach ulcers

the formation of cataracts

serious kidney complications

psychological disturbances such as depression

Unfortunately, this is only a partial list of possible side-effects associated with prolonged high doses of this powerful drug. The development of unwanted side effects from corticosteroid drugs is related to the dose of medication, how the medicine is administered and the duration of treatment. The incidence and severity of these harmful side effects can be minimized by regulating the amount of drug administered, the length of time the medication is taken, the dosage form used and the dosing schedule.

Earlier in this section, I stated my preference for using an intermediate-acting steroid such as prednisone or prednisolone over the long-acting forms like betamethasone and dexamethasone. Medical researchers have shown that forms of cortisone which are rapidly metabolized (used up) by the body are less likely to cause injury to the adrenal glands. These glands are the source of cortisone in the body and are essential for life.

Longer-acting forms of cortisone such as betamethasone and dexamethasone exert their effects on the body for two or three times longer than either prednisone and prednisolone. These long-acting drugs therefore have a greater tendency to suppress adrenal gland function.

When prescribing a cortisone preparation, I try to use the smallest dose for the shortest period that will produce the desired clinical response. The goal should always be to discontinue cortisone as soon as possible.

If steroids are used for four-to-seven-day periods and then stopped, the possibility that any long-lasting side effects will develop is extremely small. With the exception of a patient who had an increase in appetite, I cannot recall seeing anyone who has had a significant problem with a short course of cortisone.

If it becomes necessary to keep a child on longer-term cortisone therapy because of severe asthma, then the methods of choice are the use of an aerosolized preparation given three to four times a day or the oral administration of a preparation such as prednisone given as a single dose once every other morning. This is known as an alternate-day schedule. Using either of these techniques significantly reduces the incidence of harmful side effects. You should discuss these options with your child's doctor.

Table 5 Summary of Corticosteroids for use in Asthma

Oral

Prednisolone Tablets 1 mg and 5 mg white tablets.

Prednesol (soluble prednisolone) 5 mg pink scored tablets, suitable for children unwilling to swallow tablets.

Delta-Cortril (enteric coated prednisolone) 2.5 mg brown and 5 mg red tablets. Since these tablets are designed to pass through the stomach and dissolve in the intestine, gastric irritation is kept to a minimum.

Doses range up to 30 mg or more.

Injection

Hydrocortisone injection usually given by slow intravenous injection which is less painful than intra-muscular. Doses up to 100 mg reserved for serious situations as the oral route is almost as quick.

Inhalation

Becotide and Becloforte, brand names for beclomethasone MDIs

Becotide Rotacaps – 100 mg and 200 mcg.

Becotide Solution – for use in nebulizers

Bextasol – brand name for Betamethasone MDI

Pulmicort – brand name for Budesonide MDI

No other corticosteroid preparations are required to treat asthma effectively.

Monitoring steroids As yet, there is no practical way to monitor steroid levels in the blood in the way that we can monitor theophylline. If a child must use high doses of cortisone for prolonged periods of time, periodic checks of adrenal gland function may be necessary. A variety of blood tests can be used to determine whether there is any impairment of adrenal function. The need for such tests arises infrequently, and then only for children who have been on cortisone for extended periods of time.

Summary of suggestions and recommendations for the use of steroids Steroids are such potent drugs that a review of the caveats issued so far is in order. Here are your major concerns if your child's asthma is serious enough to warrant steroid treatment:

Make sure your doctor uses steroids only when they are

absoutely necessary: that is, only when other asthma drugs have been tried and have not provided adequate relief. This is the first and the last rule of steroid administration. If steroids are required, make sure that the smallest necessary dose is used for the shortest possible period of time.

I prefer to see a child receive his total twenty-four hour dose of steroids as a single morning dose. After medication is given for a four-to-seven-day course, it may then be discontinued. If cortisone is needed for more than ten to fourteen days, the dose should be gradually decreased for a period of time before being discontinued.

If it becomes necessary to give repeated short pulse doses of cortisone over a three-to-six month period, your doctor should recommend the alternate-day method of treatment. If your child is old enough to use a metered dose inhaler, an aerosolized steroid preparation is probably the safest method of administration.

Any child who has taken cortisone for a month or more will almost certainly develop some degree of adrenal gland suppression. While this condition is reversible, it may take as long as a year before adrenal gland function returns to normal. During this period, if particularly stressful circumstances occur – such as a severe infection or the need for surgery – it may be necessary to give cortisone for several days until the acute episode has passed. This procedure, I repeat, is required only for children who have used corticosteroids for long periods of time.

If the long-term use of a corticosteroid is absolutely necessary, it is the doctor's responsibility to discuss with the parents the risks involved *before* these medications are administered. Any doctor who prescribes large doses of steroids for extended periods of time without first talking it over with the family is, in my opinion, practising bad medicine.

Long-term oral steroids should be given in the lowest possible effective dose. The doctor should make every effort constantly to lower and ultimately to discontinue the use.

Steroids should be the last drug used in the treatment of chronic asthma and the first one discontinued. If your child is given steroids before first being tried on theophylline, the beta-adrenergics and sodium cromoglycate, something is wrong. Find out what it is. Perhaps a second opinion is in order. At least bring the subject to light with your doctor and ask why he is using these potent medications. If the answer does not satisfy you, and if a second opinion justifies your doubt, consider switching doctors.

What has been said refers to those steroids which are given orally or by injection, and although at first sight it is very alarming you must be willing to be guided by your doctor and not put difficulties in his way if he genuinely thinks your child needs steroids. It is possible that he sees danger signs that you do not and, in trying to save your child from the undoubted side effects of steroids, you may be opting for a course of action that puts your child in even more danger of trying to cope with a life-threatening malady. This puts the contention at its starkest, and with proper rapport between doctor and patient (or patient's parent) arguments over treatment should not arise.

What follows refers to a different class of corticosteroids, those which are inhaled: beclomethasone (Becotide and Becloforte), betamethasone in its inhaled form (Bextasol), budesonide (Pulmicort and Pulmicort IS), and Aldecin (widely used in Australia). These are either given by MDI or, in the case of Becotide (made by the same firm as Ventolin), in the dry powder Rotahaler/ Rotacap form. Becotide can also be given by nebulizer; by this inhaled route only a very minute amount is actually absorbed into the bloodstream. The bulk of the drug has its effect on the lining of the lungs and does not get into the body in the same way as steroids given by mouth or injection. Studies on the breakdown products that appear in the urine show that not enough is absorbed to produce the ill effects of steroids listed above.

As with bronchodilator drugs given by inhalation, the dose of inhaled steroids is measured in micrograms as opposed to milligrams. They can be likened to the low-strength steroid creams which are sold over the counter without prescription. They just work on the surface without being incorporated to any degree.

So, with these distinctions in mind, it can be seen that long-term administration of inhaled steroids is not dangerous. It is now becoming a standard long-term treatment and in recent months there has developed an influential school of thought amongst asthma doctors that inhaled steroids should be a first-line treatment and bronchodilators used to control episodes when the asthma 'breaks through'. It is thought that if 'twitchy airways' can be kept from reacting to allergens, after a while they become less 'twitchy' and eventually, over a period of many months, or years even, the asthmatic tendency can be lessened and possibly eliminated. This theory has become current only in the last year and there are doctors who disagree with it.

Antibiotics

Most children who wheeze in association with an upper respiratory tract infection will *not* benefit from the use of antibiotics. The reason is simple: most colds are caused by viruses, not by bacteria. Currently available antibiotics do not kill viruses, so to prescribe an antibiotic for a viral infection will accomplish very little. The only time antibiotics really earn their keep is when a serious bacterial infection such as a strep throat or ear infection is associated with the asthma. Then such a drug is clearly in order. If some question arises as to whether or not an infection is viral or bacterial, a visit to the doctor for advice is the best move.

Using antibiotics for asthma and allergies Erythromycin, an antibiotic frequently prescribed for children, may cause problems for any asthmatic youngster who is also taking theophylline. The antibiotic slows down the metabolism of theophylline, which can lead to an increased level of theophylline in the blood. In this situation, signs and symptoms of theophylline toxicity may develop. I would advise you to become familiar with these symptoms as described on page 99 and to be on the watch for them.

Questions have been raised regarding the use of penicillin for an allergic child with asthma. Currently, there is no evidence to indicate that an allergic child runs a greater risk of developing an allergic penicillin reaction than a nonallergic, nonasthmatic child.

Finally, let me repeat that under most circumstances an

asthma attack will *not* require antibiotics as part of the usual course of treatment. When a bacterial infection is associated with acute asthma symptoms, then treatment with these drugs is absolutely necessary. Unfortunately, most childhood infections, especially those involving the upper respiratory tract, are caused by viruses, against which antibiotics are of no avail. It has been my experience that only a relatively small percentage of children with acute asthma really require an antibiotic.

Expectorants

One of the major problems children have during an asthma attack is the accumulation of large amounts of thick, sticky mucus in the lungs. Expectorants are supposed to thin these secretions and make them easier to eliminate.

In theory this sounds great, but to date the pharmaceutical companies have been unable to produce any really effective expectorants. Indeed, if the truth be told, the best expectorant is plain old H_2O, though fluids in any form, hot or cold, are as effective as the commercial products you purchase from the chemist.

Antihistamines

For children unlucky enough to have both asthma and allergic rhinitis there is a lot of confusion regarding the use of antihistamines. The theoretical reason for not prescribing antihistamines is their potential to dry out the mucus in the bronchial tubes, which would worsen asthma symptoms. In practice this problem rarely occurs. In my experience, if a child is regularly taking a bronchodilator I cannot recall any situation when asthma symptoms increased after an antihistamine was taken. Recently, some evidence has been published suggesting that in some patients asthma symptoms have improved while on antihistamines. Although many antihistamines are now available without prescription, I would urge you to discuss your child's specific situation with your allergist or doctor before administering these drugs.

MANAGING THE CHILD WITH CHRONIC ASTHMA

ASTHMATIC CHILDREN AND FAMILY TRAUMA: DON'T UNDERESTIMATE THE STRAIN

Because of the time, effort and expense required to care for a child with chronic asthma, the stress parents suffer can become as severe as the child's symptoms. In my own practice I have seen marriages break up under the pressures an asthmatic child's needs and demands exert on parents. These stresses filter down through the entire family structure, disrupting life on many levels, making the simplest things difficult in a thousand ways.

For example, a long-time family pet must suddenly be given away to friends; the best explanation the parents can come up with to rationalize this seemingly cruel act is that the animal 'makes Tommy wheeze'. 'So what!' cry Tommy's brothers and sisters, and rebellion fills the air. Meanwhile, Tommy's food sensitivities turn daily kitchen activities into an uphill battle, forcing mother to prepare two separate meals, one for her asthmatic child, one for everyone else. Beloved family activities are curtailed or even ended completely: camping, antique-hunting, picnicking, ball games, dining out, visits to the zoo – all go by the board. Parents in turn become tyrannical over what were once petty concerns, screaming at their children lest they track asthma-causing dust into the house or forget to close a window. Special attention is lavished on Tommy while the needs of the other brothers and sisters – in their minds, at any rate – are neglected. On and on it goes, the pressures increasing as the asthma drags on, parents, siblings and sick child lining up one against the other in endless confrontations, all of which, it somehow seems, end up centred around poor Tommy's 'condition'.

What's the remedy? I have no cure-alls for you, but some things will definitely help.

Talking frankly about Tommy's asthma with all family members is a good starting point. Acknowledge that problems *do* exist and that everyone in the family has a part to play in eliminating or at least reducing them. Pretending, wearing rose-coloured glasses to protect the sick child and other family members, making believe that everything is just fine and that Tommy's difficulties are 'just a phase' will only make matters worse.

Agree to work together *as a family team* to make things better, both for the patient and for the entire family.

Begin by looking for alternatives to activities that the child's asthma has made impractical. If the seaside is out for holidays, try the mountains, a lakeside holiday or even a summer visit to an interesting city. If it's no longer feasible to fill your house with overstuffed antique chairs, start collecting contemporary furnishings instead. In other words, instead of nursing antagonisms over lost pleasures, be creative. Think of ways to replace them.

When an especially heavy load falls on a single family member, help out. Divide the labour and let everyone pitch in. If extra housekeeping is required to keep the dust down, if special meals must be prepared, make sure that everyone does his or her share. Such combined efforts will not only lighten everyone's labour but will provide that special satisfaction which comes from working together as a mutually caring team.

Don't be afraid to seek professional counselling if you feel you and your family need it. If pressures in an asthmatic household become too great, a visit to a therapist or family counsellor may be just what is needed. These professionals are specially trained to help in stressful situations, and you may be surprised to hear the interesting, timely and unexpected suggestions they come up with. By no means should you take such a visit as an admission of failure or as a sign that you or the child are 'sick'. Nor should you suppose that by visiting a counsellor you are roping yourself into years and years on the couch. Often, after a few open and pertinent sessions, families have received all the help they need. From then on, problems that previously seemed insurmountable are handled with relative ease.

SELF-MANAGEMENT TECHNIQUES FOR THE ASTHMATIC CHILD: HOW DO THEY WORK?

The more an asthmatic child is encouraged to manage his own condition, the better off everyone will be, including the child. By self-management I do *not* mean that your child should serve as his own doctor. Of course not. Self-management means that both the parents and the child gather as much information as possible concerning what can safely be done at home to help the asthma and that they put this information into practice, regularly and systematically, without fail.

First, talk to your doctor Get the hard facts and integrate them into your approach to your child's day-to-day welfare. Find out:

> what your child can safely do at home to manage the condition

> how you as a parent can help

> how you can learn to gauge when a situation is self-manageable and when it is not

> how to know when to call the doctor for advice

Any responsible doctor will be willing to spend time with you on these details and provide the information necessary to start a programme of successful self-management. Before you begin, make sure you are clear on all the details.

Ask questions If you don't understand something the doctor has said concerning self-management, say so. Be certain you get it all. If you are unsure why you must give your child a particular medicine every six hours or what the reason is for taking an aerosol treatment every morning, you will probably not be very effective in making sure that the job gets done. On the other hand, if you know why certain procedures must be carried out at certain times and in certain ways, you will be far more likely to follow instructions. So ask. Don't be satisfied until you feel confident in your knowledge.

Once you have a course of self-management set up, comply with it carefully One possible reason asthma attacks continue to occur among children who are under a doctor's care is that both the parents and patient do not carefully comply with his recommendations. In other words, failure to follow the daily medicine routine will inevitably encourage the development of symptoms. Common sense tells us this must be so. And while there is no guarantee that sticking to a set course of medication will always prevent such episodes from occurring, certainly *failing* to follow medical instructions is quite likely to lead to an attack.

Asthma is a condition which fluctuates by the hour, so instruction given by your doctor must contain a degree of flexibility to cope with differing circumstances. You should understand clearly the limits within which you are able to vary the prescribed medication; how much you can raise the dose without reference to the doctor; and at what point you should call him. The severity of asthma is difficult to judge just by looking at or listening to the patient. Sometimes a patient can be very severely incapacitated with little to show for it, and this can be extremely dangerous. The best way of overcoming the difficulty in judging the severity of bronchospasm is by the use of a peak flow meter. As mentioned above, cheap plastic ones are available and perfectly serviceable for home use. They provide a numerical index by which you can judge the severity of the condition, and a drop in peak flow below a certain value can give a point at which medication is changed or referral to the doctor is mandatory.

THE ACTIVE ASTHMATIC CHILD: HOW TO GO ABOUT REGULATING AN ASTHMATIC CHILD'S ACTIVITIES

In my experience, some parents tend to overprotect asthmatic children from many types of stressful activities, mental or physical, out of fear that these situations will trigger an attack. The children of such parents may eventually find themselves deprived of childhood's most essential pleasures: sports, trips to the beach, games, visits to the country, pillow fights, eating out, keeping pets, spending the night at the home of a friend. Sometimes these children are overprotected into a state of passivity or helplessness. In dealing with chronic asthma you must establish a set of guidelines appropriate to the child's particular limitations. But isn't it better that these guidelines emphasize freedoms rather than limitations? Better to think in terms of possible do's than in absolute don'ts?

To begin with, everyone – doctor, patient and parents –

should discuss *together* the limits to be placed on a child's activities. Guidelines reached through a consensus are more likely to be followed than those handed down, as it were, from above by an overbearing doctor or a set of inflexible parents.

These guidelines can be agreed upon in the doctor's surgery when everybody is present. Everyone should have a say in the matter of which sports Johnny or Susie can participate in, what toys they can or cannot keep in their room, what pets are safe to have in the house. When deciding these questions, keep one especially important rule in mind: *Base decisions on actual asthma experiences, not theoretical possibilities.* The fact that Jonathan wheezes whenever he visits a farm is no reason to suppose that young Elizabeth will do the same. Until you know for certain that Elizabeth's asthma is triggered by barnyard animals, visits to farms should be allowed.

In other words, avoid comparing your child to other asthmatic children. Each case is different, each has its own problems, each requires a separate medical strategy. Try not to generalize. The boundaries set on a child's comings and goings depend to a large extent on age, severity of asthma, and the child's ability to accept directions responsibly. The guiding factor behind it all should be allowing the most freedom possible and forbidding an activity *only* when it is proved to trigger an attack. The goal in setting limits is to work towards fewer and fewer restrictions, not more and more.

Added to these goals should be an effort to prevent asthmatic children from feeling that they are somehow being punished by the restrictions placed on them, or that the various no's and don'ts invoked for their protection are necessarily permanent. Children's minds, especially younger children's minds, work differently from those of adults. Even if their pleasures are eliminated in the high-sounding name of good health or everyone's 'best interests', most will automatically assume they have done something wrong to deserve this deprivation. When they are forced to comply with these limitations, they will feel that they are being disciplined. Make clear to the child that these measures are being taken to protect, not to punish, and that they will change and be modified as the condition itself changes. However you choose to handle this delicate situation, make it a rule never to let a child believe that the curtailment of favourite activities is either permanent or punitive.

PREPARING IN ADVANCE FOR AN ASTHMATIC ATTACK

Here it is, plain and simple: there is absolutely no doubt that the way in which parents deal with their child's asthma can have a significant effect on the severity of the attack. If a parent becomes hysterical whenever his child starts to wheeze, if the household suddenly becomes filled with excited shrieks about hospitals and oxygen masks, if a mad search ensues for the MDI and the medicine bottle, then the child will invariably pick up on the frenzy and her asthma will become accordingly intense. It simply works that way. During a severe asthmatic episode the child will look to you for strength, clear instructions and a sense of calmness. It's up to you to provide all three.

Prepare yourself for the situation in advance.

Learn the early warning signs of asthma. As soon as they appear, take the appropriate medical steps immediately. Do not wait until the attack has time to develop before giving medication. For children who have rapid onset of severe symptoms, the wearing of a Medic Alert bracelet may be appropriate in case attacks occur away from home. Have a clear plan for handling an attack. Discuss it with your doctor so that you have confidence in your ability to cope with the situation.

Keep all necessary medications, aerosol pumps, instructions, prescriptions, lists, notes, records, phone numbers (including those for the doctor, hospital and ambulance) and books pertaining to your child's asthma in a well-marked, accessible place. Running around at the onset of an attack looking for these things will only add to the confusion. Get organized beforehand and stay that way.

With careful observation, discover everything you can about the patterns and eccentricities of your child's asthma. Learn to identify the signs and symptoms of a mild asthma attack versus an asthma emergency. The more you learn and understand, the more confident you will feel next time an attack begins.

During a severe episode parents must make every effort to appear calm, confident and self-assured. Even if the attack reaches emergency proportions, panicky behaviour by the parents will only produce anxiety in the child. At such times parents must be decisive and act with confidence, even if they are uncertain and highly anxious.

Along these lines, a little mental preparation may help. Pick a time when all is calm. Sit quietly and systematically think out in advance all the steps you would take should your child have a severe attack. Go over each of these steps one by one: where the medicine is kept, how to measure the dosages, what physical signs to look for, how to get to the hospital should a trip be necessary, and so forth. Mentally rehearse this process from beginning to end, and as you do so, visualize yourself moving through it all with strength and confidence. Assuming that you practise this bit of preparatory thinking at regular intervals, it will help you to be more mentally *and* emotionally in control next time an attack arrives. Stressful situations *can* be prepared for in advance.

Call for medical assistance if you are uncertain how to proceed when an attack begins. It is good to try and determine what direction the episode is taking. If it continues to worsen after medication is given, if breathing becomes increasingly laboured, if there is a decrease in the child's ability to talk or walk, and if the danger symptoms mentioned on page 84 start to appear, then and only then are emergency tactics appropriate. Again, *knowledge* of the way your child's asthma symptoms progress is crucial.

WHEN YOUR CHILD MUST GO TO THE HOSPITAL

Unfortunately, despite our best efforts, many children each year are admitted to hospitals for the treatment of asthma which has become so severe that all outpatient treatments have failed to control the symptoms. These children are in status asthmaticus and require immediate hospitalization. At Babies' Hospital, the children's division of Columbia Presbyterian Medical Center in New York, status asthmaticus has been *the* most frequent nonsurgical reason for hospitalization. Between four and five hundred children a year are admitted for asthma treatment, and about 1 to 2 per cent of these patients are so ill that they must be admitted to the intensive care unit.

Being admitted to a hospital is an unsettling experience, to say the least. Both patient and parent may already be exhausted from sleepless nights and both will be enervated from the ordeal of the attack, which by now has gone on for many hours or even several days. Upon arriving at the hospital, instead of receiving a respite from this turmoil they will be greeted by the hectic atmosphere of the casualty department and the hurry-up-and-wait protocol at the admissions desk.

While not much can be done to make this encounter more pleasant, you can get through the admissions procedure a bit more quickly, as well as help the attending doctor get a clearer picture of your child's problem, if you come prepared to answer the following questions related to the attack:

When did the attack begin?

Was there evidence of an accompanying cold or infection?

Was there a fever?

Has there been vomiting or diarrhoea since the attack began?

Has your child been drinking fluids? Approximately how much fluid has he or she taken within the past twenty-four hours?

Exactly what medicines has the child taken and in what specific dose? At what time of day and night were they administered?

In the hospital a variety of medications may be given in an attempt to stop the attack. Which drugs are used depends on how long the episode has been in progress and the type of medications administered at home. The following drugs and procedures are frequently ordered.

The first measure commonly used in control of an acute serious asthma attack or status asthmaticus is to give a bronchodilator via a nebulizer. When asthma is severe an ordinary MDI can become ineffective or the patient cannot breathe in sufficiently strongly to transport the medication into the lungs. A nebulizer is a device which projects a high-velocity airstream through a chamber containing the medication so that it sucks it up by the Venturi principle and produces a fine mist. Ultrasonic models are also available, but these are not recommended: they are generally not so robust, more expensive and, in some cases, can precipitate a deterioration of symptoms.

Salbutamol, terbutaline, fenoterol, reproterol and ipratropium bromide can all be given by nebulizer. Often the medicament is diluted with saline as the moist mist alone has a beneficial effect on the airways, helping to dissipate sticky mucus. The mist is inhaled either through a mask or a mouthpiece. Sometimes a stream of oxygen rather than air is used to produce the mist.

Nebulizers have become much more plentiful in the last few years; many doctors have them in their surgeries or can bring them to the patient's home on visits, and a few patients whose asthma is a constant problem have them in their own homes, as they are quite simple to learn to use. This has undoubtedly cut down on admissions to hospital, but there is still the danger of patients relying too heavily on their efficiency and continuing to use them past the safe stage of an asthma attack. Before a doctor allows a nebulizer into a home to be used by the patient without his presence, he has to be very sure that all the family fully understand its limitations and its use should be under continual review, with the parents reporting on frequency of use and efficacy and being aware at what stage further help is required. Again, the plastic peak flow meters give a definite figure to relate to rather than chancy guesses as to degree of wheeze and general condition.

As well as bronchodilators, the inhaled steroid beclomethasone (Becotide) and sodium cromoglycate (Intal) can be given by nebulizer. This brings these medications into use for children too young to use an MDI, Rotahaler or Spinhaler.

IV If none of the preceding measures stops the attack, the doctor may start an intravenous infusion, commonly known as an IV, in order to administer aminophylline, a form of theophylline, and to get more fluids directly into the child's system. The needle on the IV will be inserted into the hand, foot, or in the inside part of the arm opposite the elbow. If your child has already been taking theophylline, a blood test will also be done to determine the theophylline level in the blood. This information will help the doctor to decide on the amount of theophylline to place in the IV.

ABG determination When an attack has been in progress for many hours, significant metabolic changes take place that affect the oxygen content of the blood, the carbon dioxide level, and the relationship between the body's acid and base levels. The doctor can determine if any dangerous imbalances have resulted from these changes by checking the arterial blood gases. This test requires that a blood specimen be taken from an artery and that the specimen be analysed for its oxygen content, carbon dioxide level, and acidity. Most children admitted to a hospital for asthma will require at least one ABG study and perhaps more, depending on the severity of the attack.

Chest X-ray X-rays may be used to check for the presence of infection – for example, pneumonia – or to locate areas of the lungs that have become blocked or partially collapsed (atelectasis) due to the presence of mucus plugs. In a very small number of cases, X-ray studies will also be ordered to determine if, resulting from the popping of a small air sac during an especially severe attack, air has escaped from the lungs and entered the chest cavity, a condition known as pneumomediastinum. In some cases escaped air will also penetrate into the thorax region resulting in a condition called pneumothorax; the heart area, causing pneumopericardium; or the subcutaneous tissues of the upper chest and neck regions, causing subcutaneous emphysema. The diagnosis of this last condition can be made by running the fingers along the chest and neck of the patient; the presence of free air within the tissues will produce a sound similar to that of crinkling cellophane. This condition, though bizarre, usually disappears without medical assistance. More serious are pneumothorax and pneumopericardium, both of which may cause serious compression of the lungs and the heart and are thus potentially life-threatening. Observation and treatment in an intensive care unit are required if these problems develop.

Corticosteroids Once the decision has been made to admit your child to a hospital, the preceding treatments will be given on a continuous basis. If there are no signs of improvement after a six- or twelve-hour period, your doctor may then begin a short course of steroids. Initially these drugs are given through an IV for several days. After this period of time the vast majority of children are well enough to take their medicine by mouth and are soon ready to be discharged from the hospital.

As indicated, hospitalization can be a traumatic experience for both parents and child. One way of reducing the shock is by asking questions whenever a procedure takes place that you do not understand. We all become less fearful when we know why particular things are being done to us or to our loved ones. It is your right to have this knowledge. It is your duty to ask these questions.

A FEW ADDITIONAL THOUGHTS FOR THE ASTHMATIC CHILD

Keep your child's weight under control Obesity and asthma are a bad combination for several important reasons. If your child is overweight, the excess poundage will affect his already strained ability to remain lively and to participate in games and sports. Asthma tends to make some children passive wallflowers, especially those who are pampered by their parents and of whom nothing is asked or expected. Excess weight will compound the problem.

Being overweight puts an additional strain on the heart. Owing to the increased workload placed on a youngster's cardiac system during an asthmatic episode, fatigue will develop quickly and the child will have less energy available to cope with the attack.

A patient's extra weight makes it particularly difficult for the doctor to calculate appropriate doses of asthma medications.

As most parents will agree, asthmatic youngsters often think of themselves as different from other children. Add to this already unhealthy situation the negative body image that excess weight invariably produces, and you have a double jeopardy. Whenever possible, make sure your child keeps her weight under control. Why add further problems to an already complicated situation?

Physical activity is important The point is so vital that I'll say it again: asthmatic children should be encouraged to participate in a regular programme of sports, games and age-appropriate play. I would rather see an asthmatic child take constant medication and, as a result, actively engage in athletics than take no medicine at all and stand sulkily behind the playground fence like an outcast, watching his friends have fun.

Take all the proper common-sense precautions There are many of these, some obvious, some not. If you smoke, don't do it around your child. Make sure your child gets plenty of fresh, wholesome foods, and eliminate foods you suspect may trigger attacks. When pets cause trouble, squarely face that fact and decide whether or not to place the pet elsewhere, keep it outside, or isolate it in a separate part of the house. Make sure that all responsible members of the family know how to help out with medication schedules and self-treatment methods, and be sure others are carefully trained to do this work should you for whatever reason be absent. Avoid planning holidays in areas where you *know* the child will have trouble. Don't leave medicines where they can accidentally fall into the wrong hands, and, of course, keep them away from small children at all times. Make sure you always have a generous supply of necessary medications to hand; don't wait to run out before refilling prescriptions. This is especially true when you are going away on holiday. Make sure you have an adequate supply of medicine. Alert all teachers in school to your child's condition and seek their co-operation. Keep the home environment as stable and serene as possible, and don't forget the value of a sense of humour in coping with just about *any* problem. See to it that the child understands his or her asthma, how it works, what it is, why it occurs, what to expect; the more informed a child is on this subject, the less fearful she is likely to be in time of attack.

Learn all you can about the disease The more knowledgeable every family member is regarding asthma, the more effectively the problem can be managed. Information concerning medications, how to give them, when to take them, usual and unusual side effects and so forth should be acquired, along with a general understanding of what causes asthma.

Your primary information resource is, of course, your doctor. After taking what you can from this source, go to the library, where you'll find many books on allergies and asthma. The Asthma Research Council and the Asthma Society and Friends of the Asthma Research Council are situated at 300 Upper Street, London N1 2XX, telephone 01–226 2260. They spread knowledge about asthma and publish a number of informative leaflets and books. By joining the Asthma Society you will be eligible for a regular copy of *Asthma News* and your subscription will go towards research into asthma. There are over 100 branches throughout Britain. In some places there are local Asthma Societies attached to hospitals which operate independently of the central organization. For more information, see Appendix.

QUESTIONS AND ANSWERS ABOUT ASTHMA

Must an asthmatic child take medicine even when there are no obvious signs of wheezing or shortness of breath?

It depends on the child's particular condition. Bronchodilator drugs, discussed earlier in this chapter, should be taken for at least four to six days after all obvious symptoms of acute asthma have disappeared. Continuing the medicine will permit the patient's lungs to return to a more normal functional level. After this period of time, assuming that all the youngster's symptoms have disappeared, these drugs can be discontinued. If, on the other hand, a child's attacks occur at such frequent intervals that she is never comfortable for more than two or three days at a time, this child is clearly a chronic sufferer. In such a case I would recommend the use of bronchodilators on a daily schedule basis.

Sodium cromoglycate (Intal) should be used when there is no wheeze. Remember it is a prophylactic or preventative measure; when the wheeze has started it is really too late so Intal, in some cases, is used continuously, wheeze or no wheeze. As mentioned above, there is the new tendency to use inhaled steroids on a continuous basis to reduce the 'twitchiness' of airways.

How exactly do you define 'chronic' asthma?

There is probably no single definition agreed on by all doctors. I feel that if a child has suffered repeated attacks of asthma for longer than one year, his case can be described as chronic. At the same time there is, as in most things, also a matter of degree in any chronic condition, and this may be determined by looking at several revealing variables:

How frequent are the attacks?

How prolonged are the attacks?

How severe are the attacks?

Are the attacks becoming more intense or less intense?

Are the attacks becoming more common or less common?

For example, any child who wheezes several times a week for a period of six months to a year can certainly be said to have chronic asthma. But you might also look at a child who has wheezed only two or three times a year over the past four or five years and also say that, technically, this case is chronic. The two situations are clearly quite different, and I would manage each in an entirely different way: medication on a regular basis for the first situation, medication only during those periods when the child becomes symptomatic in the second. Yet both are technically chronic.

How should an asthmatic child be prepared before undergoing elective surgery?

With our present knowledge and the anti-asthma medications available, the potential problems surgery may entail can be avoided.

Your child should be examined by his or her regular doctor in the week before the scheduled operation. At that time a decision will be made regarding which medication, if any, has to be prescribed. If the child's lungs are not completely clear, then a three-to-five-day course of prednisone (cortisone) in addition to

an oral bronchodilator should be given. If any cortisone preparation has been taken within six months of the surgery date, it is
advisable for your child to have a short (three-to-five-day) course
of an appropriate short-acting steroid.

At the time of the operation the anaesthetist, who will be
aware of your child's asthma history, will use the anaesthetic least
likely to aggravate or trigger asthma symptoms.

After surgery, special attention will be given to your child
to prevent the development of an asthma attack. These steps may
include the use of intravenous aminophylline, an aerosolized bronchodilator, and possibly steroids. The child will be encouraged to
do some simple breathing exercises and to cough regularly to
prevent the accumulation of large amounts of mucus in the lungs.

Today, if your child needs some type of surgery, the fact
that he or she has asthma is rarely reason for added concern.

**What is the ideal geographic environment for an asthmatic child?
What parts of the country are best for this condition?**

There is no ideal environment for a person with asthma, just
as there is no typical asthmatic child. As to safe and unsafe parts
of the country, whenever consideration of a move from one
geographic area to another is contemplated, there is no way of
predicting how such a move will affect the child. Most short-term
changes of residence do prove beneficial, but usually only in the
beginning. Problems come later on, six months or a year after the
move is made. The local pollens, the local air pollution, the local
animals, the local allergens all take their toll, and things may be
back where they started. Moving solely to escape an allergy is a
risky business at best and has no proven medical benefits.

What role does air pollution play in asthma?

There is no question that air pollution of any type – whether
from car exhausts, industrial contamination or unusual weather
patterns – can have a harmful effect on most asthmatics. The
irritating action on the lungs of various chemical compounds such
as sulphur dioxide and carbon monoxide have been responsible for
triggering many acute attacks. At best, these chemical irritants

aggravate pre-existing asthma conditions; in a small but identifiable percentage of patients they may be the cause of the asthma. There are specific indoor-work-related situations in which employees who have been chronically exposed to excessive levels of toxic chemicals develop symptoms of asthma. Some preliminary information suggests that in homes equipped with gas ovens and cooking ranges children with asthma tend to have more symptoms. This early observation is being evaluated in a number of current research projects. In short, both indoor and outdoor air pollution can and in many instances does play a definable role.

Does cigarette smoke bother asthma?

Absolutely and unquestionably. Tobacco smoke is a primary irritant for *anyone* with asthma. It is harmful just to be in a room where cigarette smoke is hanging in the air. As for adolescent asthmatics who take up the cigarette habit, all any doctor can say to them is this: PLEASE STOP NOW! RIGHT NOW! before any real damage is done and before the addiction becomes permanent.

Is there any proof that asthmatic children suffer from emotional problems more frequently than nonasthmatic children?

From my own experience and from most of the evidence we have today, there seem to be no identifiable psychological differences between children with asthma and children without. Among youthful asthma sufferers you will find all personality types, all physical types, all psychological types, all social types – there is no 'typical' asthmatic child. Many people have claimed that asthmatic children are loners, preferring their own company to that of others; or that such children are introverted, brooding, even emotionally unstable. I think that children who suffer from any chronic medical problem that keeps them socially isolated from other children and singles them out as strange or different will invariably become a bit withdrawn. In other words, I do not believe it is the personality of the child that contributes to the asthma, but the condition of being asthmatic that affects the personality. Proof of this in my own practice has come from observing the occasional withdrawn child with chronic severe asthma become an outgoing, actively participating member of his social group as his condition is brought under control.

> At one time many professionals claimed that 'smother love' – i.e., an overbearing, overprotective and overcontrolling attitude on the part of the mother – was a major contributing factor in the development of asthma. Is this theory still given credence?

The whole question of the psychological relationship of the parents to the child, and specifically the mother to the child, vis-à-vis the development of asthma, is an issue that has simply never been settled one way or the other. Some years ago, in an attempt to establish a definite link between asthma and the emotions, psychologists and psychiatrists developed a psychological type they called the asthmatic personality. One of the identifying traits of this type was a domineering mother. The concept has not stood the test of time, and the final verdict is that evidence for its support is inconclusive at best.

> Do you recommend the use of relaxation techniques such as biofeedback, meditation, hypnosis or autohypnosis for help with asthma?

Any relaxation technique that can help to relieve the anxiety and emotional stress associated with an asthma attack is worth trying. I have been impressed with the lessening of symptoms some patients have exhibited with the use of biofeedback and self-hypnosis. Providing that the patient receives proper instruction from a qualified professional, I have no objection to a trial with these techniques. Breathing exercises can be useful techniques for relaxation.

CHAPTER SIX

Chronic Rhinitis

Christopher, aged nine, is in good health and is a perfectly normal, happy youngster except for a single recurring problem: each year in early spring he begins to sneeze, has a constantly runny nose, and complains of itchy eyes and throat. Like clockwork, these bothersome symptoms start up some time in April and continue without a break through to early July.

Janet, aged thirteen, has had a two-year history of nasal congestion. Her problem surfaces in late October when the forced-air heating in her home is turned on, and continues until early spring. Her father is pondering the unpleasant prospect of replacing the entire household heating system.

Angela, aged five, has been in nursery school since she was three. There she experiences what appears to be a constant cold with dripping nose, cough and violent sneezing. These symptoms start in September when school begins and continue throughout the school year. Angela's teachers sometimes send her home for fear that other children in the class will catch her 'cold', but her parents know better. She, like the others, is a victim of chronic rhinitis.

These three youngsters are representative of a veritable army of children who suffer from a wide range of symptoms, all of which are lumped under a single heading: chronic rhinitis, or as a variety of it is known, hay fever. About four million people each year suffer during the summer with so-called hay fever and another two million suffer throughout the year with perennial rhinitis. Many school days are lost, the height of the hay-fever season seems to coincide with the most important exams children take, and the expense in drugs and loss of work is considerable. The bill for drugs increases every year. While clearly not a life-threatening disorder, rhinitis is responsible for significant personal and economic hardships. It is not, as the worn joke reminds us, something to be sneezed at.

INSIDE THE NASAL LABYRINTH

Before details on the different forms of rhinitis that may plague your child are provided, some background on the workings of the nose are in order. Several facts are, of course, obvious. We breathe through our nose, and our sense of smell is located in our nose. It is, however, not entirely accurate to say that this organ serves simply as a breathing tube or as a conduit for odours. In reality, our nose 'processes' air as well as drawing it in. It filters the air, humidifies it, and regulates its temperature. If these functions are not performed properly we become quite uncomfortable. Sometimes we get downright ill.

Major landmarks to become familiar with here are the three turbinates, extending from the nostrils to the nasopharynx at the back of the throat (see Figure 5). There is an *inferior* turbinate, a *middle* turbinate and a *superior* turbinate.

Look below the inferior turbinate. Here you will see the opening of the passageway connecting the nose with the eye, the nasolacrimal duct. Near it is the middle turbinate, which covers the entrances to the frontal, anterior ethmoid und maxillary sinuses, while beneath the superior turbinate you will find the opening to the posterior ethmoid and the sphenoid sinuses. Finally, the openings of the eustachian tube, which connect the ear and the nasopharynx, are situated directly behind the inferior turbinate.

All the sinuses pictured in Figure 5 drain into the nose, and this is very significant. If for some reason there is a marked swelling of the nasal tissues, either from infection, irritation or allergic reaction, the openings of these sinuses can become plugged and blocked in response. Then you have trouble. One of the primary causes for such swelling is hay fever; thus sinus problems and rhinitis not infrequently go hand in hand.

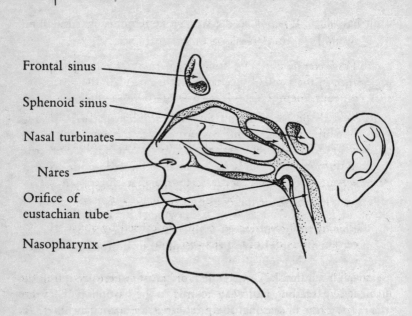

Figure 5   Cross-section of a normal nose

RHINITIS: WHAT IS IT?

Rhinitis and sinus problems are not the same thing. The first can lead to the second, but they are decidedly two different conditions. Rhinitis means an inflammation of the mucous membranes of the nose. The condition is brought about by an allergic response, an infection or a chronic irritation of the nasal mucous membranes.

While symptoms from different causes of rhinitis may appear similar – runny nose, sneezing, and nasal irritation – it is none the less crucial for the doctor to differentiate between these look-alike conditions, as treatment may vary depending on the specific diagnosis. The major forms of rhinitis your child may develop include:

Seasonal allergic rhinitis. More commonly known as hay fever.

Perennial allergic rhinitis. Like hay fever but with year-round symptoms rather than seasonal ones.

Vasomotor rhinitis. This condition is caused by an imbalance in the control mechanisms that regulate the nasal mucous membranes. It is a year-round nonallergic, noninfectious form of chronic rhinitis. The nasal membranes are stimulated to overreact to such conditions as temperature changes, irritating odours and even emotional stress.

Infectious rhinitis. Another term for upper respiratory tract infections or the common cold.

Rhinitis medicamentosa. A condition caused by abuse of certain kinds of nose drops and sprays.

Seasonal allergic rhinitis Grass pollens are most numerous during the hay-making season (mid-May to mid-July in Britain). They are the major cause of seasonal allergies; hence the name hay fever. As the grass pollens die down in mid-summer the moulds and fungi become more important as a source of allergy. The prevalence of allergens varies in different parts of the country. The seaside is often a good place for hay-fever sufferers. Paradoxically, the centres of cities are no refuge; very high pollen counts are recorded in Central London with no hay field within miles.

Chart 1 gives the times of appearances of the most common allergens in Britain.

Recognizing allergic rhinitis Clinically speaking, parents should suspect their child is suffering from seasonal allergic rhinitis if a recurring pattern of the following symptoms appears each spring, summer or early autumn:

violent sneezing spells

itching, streaming eyes

watery, clear, nonirritating nasal discharge

nasal congestion, nose itching and rubbing

Chart 1

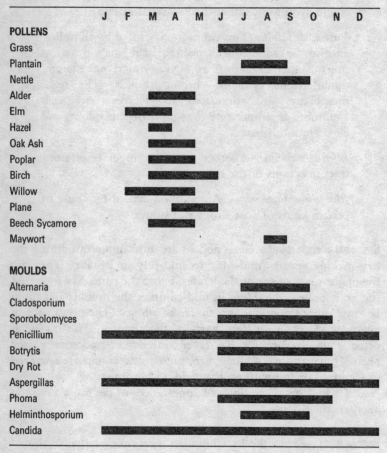

reduction in the sense of smell (mostly in older children)

mouth breathing and clearing of the throat

complaints of itching in the ears, mouth and throat

dark circles under the eyes during the allergic season

Keep an eye out for so-called colds that seem never to clear up. A child who suffers from these symptoms is probably the victim of allergic rhinitis rather than an infection. Table 6 provides a comparison of symptoms of the two conditions, infectious rhinitis (colds) and allergic rhinitis.

Children suffering from hay fever are especially prone to listlessness, moodiness and a kind of free-floating irritability. They may pick at their food, find fault with the world and generally become miserable to live with. When this mood descends, it is the parent's job to recognize that the change is due to a remedial physical problem and not to something intrinsically negative in the child's character. A trial period of four to seven days on an over-the-counter antihistamine or decongestant preparation is a reasonable way to deal with the problem. Examples of nonprescription drugs that may be effective include: Dimetane (an antihistamine), Chlortrimeton (an antihistamine), Sudafed (a decongestant), Afrinol (a long-acting decongestant), and Benadryl (an antihistamine).

Table 6   Distinguishing Hay Fever from Colds

Symptom	Allergic rhinitis	Upper Respiratory Tract Infection (URI)
Nasal discharge	Thin, watery, clear, nonirritating	Thick, yellow to green in colour; local irritation
Fever	None	Low-grade
Itching	In ears, nose, throat	Rarely present
Sneezing	Common in 'spells'	Occasional
Nasal mucous membranes	Appear pale and swollen	Reddened 'angry' looking
Personality change	Irritable, cranky, primarily local complaints	Fatigue, generalized discomfort
Duration	Weeks to months	7 to 10 days

Follow carefully the dosage instructions printed on the package. These instructions are usually on the conservative side; up to a few years ago many over-the-counter antihistamines were prescription-only drugs. If your child's symptoms disappear while he is on the medication, no additional evaluation or treatment may be necessary. If the symptoms persist or if your child cannot tolerate these preparations, then discuss the situation with your doctor.

Other forms of rhinitis: how to distinguish one from another Chronic complaints of a runny or stuffy nose along with sneezing, itching of the eyes, nose or throat; a decreased sense of taste or smell and fatigue – all these symptoms may be caused by an allergy, recurring infection or vasomotor rhinitis. At times it is not an easy task for the doctor to decide why Jenny or Jack is feeling so miserable!

Perennial allergic rhinitis The symptoms of perennial rhinitis and seasonal rhinitis (mentioned above) are the same, but perennial rhinitis is active year-round, not just during a particular pollen season. The symptoms are triggered by nonseasonal as well as seasonal allergens; dust, animal danders, wool and feathers are just a few of the many examples. One young girl I treated developed perennial rhinitis from contact with her parakeet; another from the mould spores that grew in her father's plant nursery. In general, antihistamines and decongestants may provide fairly good symptom control for most sufferers. If you detect a direct link between the cause of the problem – the parakeet, the moulds – and the symptoms, all the better. Very careful observation may, however, be necessary to find a link. Keeping the child away from the cause of the symptoms is by far the best form of treatment. The child suspected of having perennial allergic rhinitis should be evaluated with the same methods used for the patient who has seasonal rhinitis.

Vasomotor or nonallergic rhinitis This condition is neither allergic nor infectious; it develops because of an apparent imbalance of the neurological control mechanisms that regulate the nasal mucous membranes. These nerves control the very rich collection of blood vessels within the nose. If these autonomic nerves are stimulated by such challenges as changes in air temperature and humidity levels, strong, irritating odours, tobacco smoke or emotional stress, then blood flow in the nose will significantly decrease, which results in congestion of the nasal mucous membranes. Vasomotor rhinitis should be suspected when:

> Nasal symptoms occur intermittently throughout the year and there is no detectable pattern of symptoms.

The most frequent complaints are nasal congestion or watery nasal discharge.

Sneezing or itching of the eyes, ears and throat are generally absent.

Sudden changes in humidity, air pressure and temperature (i.e. going from indoor to outdoors) aggravate the nasal congestion.

Strong odours, paints, perfumes, dust and cigarette smoke provoke obvious discomfort.

The treatment of vasomotor rhinitis is especially frustrating because for many people the medicines currently available are not particularly effective in relieving their symptoms of congestion and postnasal drip. Despite this situation it is still reasonable to try various antihistamines. They seem to be effective for some children. Over-the-counter decongestants such as pseudoephedrine or phenylpropanolamine as well as prescription drugs may also be given. Finally, if none of these preparations seems to bring relief, a nasal steroid spray such as Nasalide, Beconase or Vancenase can be prescribed by your doctor. One word of caution: follow the directions for use of these steroid sprays. Don't attempt to self-medicate your child without specific direction from your doctor.

Infectious rhinitis Infectious rhinitis is primarily the result of a viral infection; in fact, it is the same as the common cold. (For a full description of the symptoms accompanying this ailment, see Table 6, page 151.) Infectious rhinitis is present if:

The symptoms last no longer than seven to ten days.

There is, in addition to nasal congestion, a nasal discharge which varies from quite thin to very thick. This discharge is usually yellow to green.

The nasal secretions are quite irritating, often causing the nostrils and upper lip to become red and raw.

Other symptoms such as a cough, fever, redness of

the inner nose, stomach upset and general malaise may accompany the nasal symptoms.

Antihistamines and decongestants can provide some relief, but not as much as might be expected with allergic rhinitis.

Rhinitis medicamentosa There is yet another variety of rhinitis, one produced by causes somewhat different from the others. Not infrequently, in an attempt to relieve a cold or an allergic nasal condition, over-the-counter decongestant nose drops or sprays may be used for many weeks at a time. Prolonged application of these drugs is an abuse, and when this occurs the medication which is supposed to control symptoms ends up making them a good deal worse. As the effectiveness of the decongestant declines and the symptoms become increasingly severe, the patient, in the true mode of the addict, comes to depend on larger and larger doses to get relief from symptoms now being caused by the drug rather than the original condition. This is known as rhinitis medicamentosa. Freely translated, the name means 'The medicine did it'.

Here is a typical scenario: Amy has a runny nose and is constantly sniffing. Her mother goes to the chemist and selects one of the many brands of nonprescription nose drops or sprays on display. This medicine is given according to the instructions on the label and at first it seems to decrease, if not entirely eliminate, Amy's congestion. After four or five days it seems that the drops must be given more frequently because the symptomatic relief Amy experiences has become increasingly shorter. Before too long, Amy's mother is giving her child doses of the spray twice a day, then four times, then eight, then in desperation ten, then more. And still the condition refuses to improve.

What to do? Simple. Throw the nose drops or sprays into the dustbin *immediately*! Unless medication is halted on the spot the symptoms will continue to worsen, and the possibility of permanent damage to the child's nasal mucous membranes will increase proportionately. Some time ago a nineteen-year-old pregnant woman who had been suffering from chronic nasal congestion for almost two years came to my consulting room. Despite medication, her condition was getting worse all the time. When I asked what drugs she was using, she dug into her handbag and produced an over-the-counter nasal spray, announcing that she had been going through a bottle of this medicine *every two days* and that she had been following this regime for *eighteen consecutive months*. The woman, it turned out, was addicted to her decongestant. The only way to get her 'unhooked' was to substitute a cortisone nasal spray for the present medication, and even then the weaning process was slow and difficult. Moral: never use over-the-counter nasal preparations carelessly, and *never* use them for more than four or five days at a time. If your child shows any signs of becoming dependent on such preparations, even when they are employed only occasionally, discontinue their use right away and consult your doctor.

TREATMENT FOR RHINITIS

Once a diagnosis has been reached based on history, physical findings and appropriate laboratory tests, recommendations for your child's rhinitis condition will be made. As with the other conditions we have discussed, treatment falls into three broad headings: pharmacotherapy, environmental control measures and immunotherapy.

PHARMACOTHERAPY

While most people associate the symptomatic treatment of allergic rhinitis with antihistamines and decongestants alone, a relatively new prophylactic agent, sodium cromoglycate, known commercially as Rynacrom, and several cortisone nasal preparations are important players on the therapeutic team. Let's have a look at these medications in more detail.

Antihistamines

When we refer to an antihistamine, we are actually speaking of six different chemical groups within the same pharmaceutical family, all of them possessing antihistamine properties. What exactly are these properties?

Antihistamines neutralize the effects of histamine, the chemical mediator responsible for causing many of the typical symptoms associated with allergy. They do this by blocking areas called receptor sites located on the surface of cells. If histamine, which is responsible for the sneezing, itchy eyes and runny nose of chronic rhinitis, is prevented from reaching these receptor sites, effective symptom control can be accomplished.

An important point to remember in this process is that anti-histamines work best *before* the histamine is released into the blood: that is, before the allergic reaction has started; and this is clearly the most efficient way to take this medicine – before the symptoms begin. (For more detailed information regarding the workings of histamine, see page 21.) Antihistamines are a rather diverse collection of drugs divided into six different groups of families. Since a drug from one of these families may be effective in providing relief for one child but not for another, your doctor may try several different varieties of antihistamine before the best one is found. Once the most effective medication is determined, it can then be used for extended periods.

A few notes on the antihistamines Liquid antihistamines are absorbed into the bloodstream rapidly and tend to go to work faster than either capsules or tablets. Whenever there is an urgent need for an antihistamine, the liquid form is your best bet.

Small children have difficulty swallowing tablets and capsules. For those under two, liquid antihistamines are the preferred form.

If your child requires daily doses of an antihistamine for an extended period of time, a long-acting tablet or capsule is the best form in which to administer the drug. Common sense tells us that taking medicine twice a day is a more efficient method of drug delivery than dosing it every six hours or four times a day.

When beginning a course of antihistamines, be alert to the development of side effects. While drowsiness is the most common, it is often mild and tends not to interfere with the child's normal functioning. If extreme drowsiness or any other side effects become a problem, discontinue the medicine and contact your doctor immediately. He will most likely switch your child to another antihistamine.

Over a period of weeks to months some children may develop a tolerance for a certain antihistamine. When this occurs, the medication will no longer be effective and another must be substituted. Armed with this knowledge, you should not be surprised if your doctor changes antihistamine prescriptions, as this switching is a normal part of rhinitis therapy. Interestingly enough, after some time has passed the child may then return to the original antihistamine and discover that it again works as well as it did before the medicine was switched.

Despite what some people may tell you, there is no one 'best' antihistamine. The best antihistamine is the one that works best for your child. Period.

Table 7 gives an overview of how antihistamine drugs are organized. The possible side effects of all these drugs include sleepiness, gastrointestinal upset, a jittery feeling, and sometimes hyperactivity.

Decongestants

Decongestants are vasoconstricting agents; this means they cause a narrowing of the blood vessels in the nasal mucous membranes which decreases the swelling and congestion found in most forms of rhinitis. These medicines can cause unpleasant side effects; children using them must be carefully watched. Specific decongestant agents include pseudoephedrine hydrochloride, ephedrine, phenylpropanolamine, pseudoephedrine SO_4 and phenylepherine. Decongestants are available in a variety of forms including liquids, tablets, nasal sprays and drops. They are often combined with an antihistamine into a single preparation, as shown in Table 8.

Among decongestants, the nose drops and spray forms are the most frequently used and abused. Therefore both for children and parents, *never use a decongestant spray or nose drops for longer than five days in a row*.

Why? Recall the pregnant woman who was addicted to decongestants. After four or five days, most topical decongestants' effective duration of action decreases considerably, so that the medicine must be administered at shorter and shorter intervals to bring relief. Eventually, through what is called a rebound mechanism, the drops or sprays begin to *cause* the nasal congestion the decongestant was designed to inhibit; at the same time the user becomes increasingly dependent on the drug, using greater and greater amounts to achieve ever less and less relief. This condition, as mentioned, is called rhinitis medicamentosa. Treatment consists of discontinuing topical nasal preparations immediately. In other words, if five or more days of use have already elapsed, throw away those drops and sprays *right now*.

Side effects In general, decongestant sprays and drops cause fewer general or systemic side effects than orally administered decongestants. When side effects do occur, typical symptoms include:

nausea

dizziness

nervousness

tachycardia (rapid heartbeat)

hyperactive behaviour

transient (temporary) high or low blood pressure, and/ or irregular heartbeat (such reactions are unusual and are generally limited to young children; stopping the medicine immediately will cause these reactions to cease)

Sodium Cromoglycate: Rynacrom and Opticrom

Sodium cromoglycate has the unique ability to block allergic reactions *before* they occur. If it worked for every patient, I could spend all my time writing books because no one would visit my consulting room with allergic symptoms. Unfortunately, for allergy sufferers there is no single drug currently available that comes even close to being 100 per cent effective, sodium cromoglycate included. Still, this useful medication is the first example of a prophylactic drug for rhinitis or conjunctivitis, and the good news is that researchers tell us that others will soon follow.

Table 7 Antihistamines

Generic names	Brand Name	Available forms
OXYETHYLAMINE TYPE		
Diphenydramine	Benadryl	Capsules
ETHYLENE DAIMINE TYPE		
Mepyramone maleate	Anthisan	Tablets
ARYLALKYLAMINE TYPE		
Triprolodine	Actidil	Tablets, elixir.
	Pro-actidil	Sustained released tablet
Pheniramine maleate	Daneral-SA	Sustained-release tablet
Chlorpheniramine	Piriton	Tablets, syrup, spandets, injection
Brompheniramine	Dimotane LA	Sustained-release tablets, tablets, elixir
Clemastine	Tavegil	Tablets, elixir
PHENIDENE TYPE		
Mebhydrolin	Fabahistin	Tablets, suspension
Phenindamine	Thephorin	Tablets
Dimethindene maleate	Fenostil Retard	Sustained-release tablet
PIPERIDENE TYPE		
Azatadine maleate	Optimine	Tablets, syrup
Diphenylpyraline	Histyl Spansule	Sustained-release capsule
	Lergoban	Sustained-release tablet.
Cyproheptadine	Periactin	Tablet, syrup
PHENOTHIAZINE TYPE		
Promethazine	Phenergan	Tablet, elixir, injection
Trimepraxine	Vallergan	Tablet, syrup
New Anthistamines		
Non-sedative Astemizole	Hismanal	Tablet, suspension
Terfenadine	Triludan	Tablet, suspension
PIPERAZINE TYPE		
Oxatomide	Tinset	Tablet
Hydroxyzine	Atarax	Tablet, syrup

Two forms of sodium cromoglycate are available for the prevention of allergic eye and nasal symptoms: Opticrom and Rynacrom. Both must be used four times a day at the beginning of treatment, either one drop of Opticrom in each eye or one spray of Rynacrom in each nostril. Clinical benefits from this drug may be detected as early as three to four days after treatment has started, or as late as the third or fourth week. When there is a positive response, the dosage can then be decreased to three times and perhaps even twice a day. Sodium cromoglycate does not relieve symptoms once they are present; it must be used on a daily basis before problems arise.

Side effects Sodium cromoglycate has been proved an extremely safe preparation that can be administered on a regular basis for long periods of time. The potential side effects, though usually minimal, may include:

sneezing

transient burning of the nasal mucous membranes

headaches

a bad taste in the mouth

These symptoms, when they do occur, are generally not serious and tend to disappear when the medication is discontinued. Really, the major problem with sodium cromoglycate is less one of side effects and more one of compliance and human error; even the most efficient parents sometimes forget to make sure their children take the drug on a regular four-times-a-day schedule, and the children themselves either cannot be bothered or are incapable of medicating themselves. Yet without faithful adherence to the recommended treatment directions, sodium cromoglycate will simply not work effectively.

What's more, while treatment is advisable for any child suffering from vasomotor or allergic rhinitis, it by no means works for everyone, and only after a period of at least four weeks can a decision be made regarding its effectiveness for your child. If your child is about to start using sodium cromoglycate look upon the chances of success with bright optimism but not with blind hope.

Table 8 Antihistamine Decongestant Overview

Name	Available	Antihistamine	Decongestant
Actifed	OTC*	Tripolodine HC1	Pseudoephedrine HC1
Benylin Decongestant	OTC	Diphenydramine HC1	Pseudoephedrine HC1
Congesteze Tablets	POM†	Azatadine Maleate	Pseudoephedrine sulphate
Congesteze Syrup	POM	Azatadine Maleate	Pseudoephedrine sulphate
Congesteze Paed. Syrup	OTC	Azatadine Maleate	Pseudoephedrine sulphate
Dimotapp Elixir	OTC	Brompheniramine Maleate	Phenylephrine HC1 Phenylpropanolamine HC1
Dimotapp Paed. Elixir	OTC	Maleate	Phenylpropanolamine HC1
Dimotapp La Tablets	OTC	Maleate	Phenylpropanolamine HC1
Eskornade Slow-Release Capsule/ Spansule	OTC	Diphenylpryaline HC1	Phenylpropanolamine
Eskornade Syrup	OTC	Diphenylpryaline HC1	Phenylpropanolamine HC1
Expurhin Paed. Linctus	OTC	Chlorpheniramine Maleate	Ephedrine HC1
Haymine Slow-Release Tablet	OTC	Chlorpheniramine Maleate	Ephedrine HC1
Rinurel Tablet	OTC	Phenyltoloxamine Citrate	Phenylpropanolamine HC1
Triominic Tablet	OTC	Pheniramine Maleate	Phenylpropanolamine HC1

* OTC = Over the counter
† POM = Prescription-only medicine

Table 9 Commonly Used Nasal Decongestants

Generic Name	Brand Name	Available Form
Pseudoephedrine HC1	Sudafed	Tablet, elixir
	Galpseud	Tablet
Oxymetazoline	Afrazine	Spray, drops
Xylometazoline	Otrivine	Spray, drops, paediatric drops
	Otrivine-Antistin	Spray, drops
Phenylephrine	Hayphryn	Spray
	Neophryn	Spray, drops

	Generic Drugs	
Xylometazoline		Nasal drops
Xylometazoline		Nasal drops paediatric
Ephedrine		Nasal drops 0.5% and 1%

NOTE: Neither drops nor sprays should be used for more than five days; then the decongestant *must* be discontinued.

Steroids

These drugs, which are derived from powerful, naturally occurring hormones produced by the adrenal glands, are potent anti-inflammatory agents. They are highly effective for the treatment of chronic rhinitis because of their ability to decrease local swelling. Their major drawback is the fact that when used for a prolonged period they can produce serious and in some situations even life-threatening side effects. They are in effect the proverbial double-edged sword.

Any steroid taken by mouth in large doses for weeks at a time will cause unwanted complications. Fortunately, within the past five years, two typically active, poorly absorbed cortisone derivatives, beclomethasone dipropionate and flunisolide, have become commercially available. These drugs are marketed as: Beconase (beclomethasone dipropionate), which comes in a gas-propelled dispenser, and Syntaris (flunisolide), which is in a pump-spray container.

Either of these preparations can be used for weeks at a time in the appropriately prescribed dose without fear of dangerous side effects. Two complaints that occur with some frequency are a transient burning sensation immediately after using the spray and, less often, the development of a bloody nose. If either of these situations develops, contact your doctor right away for new instructions. Beconase has been recommended for children down to the age of six and Syntaris down to the age of five.

For any child who continues to have significant rhinitis symptoms despite treatment with antihistamines, decongestants and sodium cromoglycate a trial with either of these cortisone derivatives is in order. Discuss the appropriate starting dose with your doctor.

A treatment for chronic rhinitis among ear, nose and throat specialists is a procedure involving injection of a long-acting steroid preparation directly into the nasal turbinates. *This technique can on rare occasions cause extremely dangerous side effects.* Given the fact that efficient topically active steroid preparations and/or quick bursts of oral steroids are available for children suffering from severe rhinitis, it is my opinion that the use of nasal steroid injections should be discouraged, if not abandoned entirely. If a doctor suggests such a procedure for your child I advise that you get a second opinion before consenting.

ENVIRONMENTAL CONTROL MEASURES

The easiest, cheapest, most painless way to relieve allergic symptoms is simply to remove the substance and/or allergen responsible for causing the problem – provided, of course, you have the luxury of knowing what the substance is. If you do, then you can practise the simplest anti-allergy measure of all: environmental control. Henry's runny nose, weeping eyes and itchy throat are, we know, due to a family cat. You can solve the problem quickly by removing the cat from the premises. A horsehair sofa makes Judy sneeze and sniffle. Replace it with a couch filled with a nonallergenic stuffing. Feathers are Larry's nemesis. Give that pet bird away to a friend or relative and get rid of all down quilts and pillows. In many cases it really is just as easy as that. Here are some practical steps you can take in this direction.

Humidification When the heating is on and especially if a forced-air form of heating is used, the air becomes exceedingly dry and irritating to the nose, mouth and throat. This dryness bothers just about everyone but is especially troublesome for children with chronic nasal congestion. In a house with low relative humidity (less than 35 per cent) a sleeping child who is a mouth breather will awaken with complaints of a sore throat. Typically, this problem is worse on arising and improves dramatically as the day progresses, only to recur the next morning! The problem stems not from a virus or a bacteria, but from a simple lack of adequate humidity in the air.

The remedy is simple: increase the amount of water vapour in the air. The optimal relative humidity for your home is between 35 and 45 per cent, and you can raise it to this level by a variety of means. One no-frills method is simply to fill pans with water and place them near the heating units in every room. The passive evaporation of the water will soon increase the level of the relative humidity in the air and your child should quickly feel the difference.

More sophisticated are the various electronic humidifiers and vaporizers on the market today. The most efficient of these is the *ultrasonic cool mist humidifier*. This space-age appliance uses sound waves to produce a superfine vapour of mist that remains suspended in the air for a long time. This humidifier manufactures water droplets so small they easily penetrate deep into a child's mouth, throat and lungs. A fringe benefit of the ultrasonic humidifier is that the water vapour is so finely dispersed throughout the atmosphere that floors, walls and bedding do not end up being drenched; the older models are not always so obliging. Sounds too good to be true? Well, there is one significant drawback: cost. The usual retail price for this machine is from £40 to £100. Not cheap. Still, careful shoppers will look for ultrasonic humidifiers on sale at the end of the summer season. As these units become increasingly popular, market competition will no doubt work its magic and drive the prices down to a more generally affordable level.

A word on steam vaporizers: while useful for children who suffer from croup and sinusitis, these devices are, in my experience, practically worthless as far as rhinitis is concerned. Hot-air vaporizers may stimulate the growth of allergy-causing moulds in and around the child's living area, and in some instances the warm steam from these appliances irritates rather than soothes the rhinitis. Similarly, there is no medical reason that I know of for adding inhalants such as eucalyptus, Vicks Vaporub and menthol to a vaporizer. Though these substances bring a pleasing medicinal odour to the immediate atmosphere and perhaps create the illusion that they are 'cleaning out' the lungs, in truth they serve no therapeutic purpose.

Dust control Dust is the accumulation of the breakdown products of all the organic materials found in the home. The dust in my home will be different from the dust in your home, depending on how each is furnished and the life-style of its occupants. A family that owns several pets, likes to keep its windows open, and has wool carpeting throughout the house will have a substantially different type of dust from the folks next door who use central air conditioning, keep no pets and have synthetic-fibre carpets.

Chief, perhaps, of all the allergens in dust is the so-called dust mite, a microscopically tiny creature that lives in every house, specifically in every bed. Unlike bedbugs, dust mites are not limited to homes of poor hygiene or poverty. Comfortably ensconced in pillows and mattresses, this ubiquitous animal derives its nourishment from the dead skin cells that flake off our bodies during the hours of rest. Vacuuming the mattress and mattress cover when the bed linen is changed and putting your pillows in a clothes dryer every few weeks will significantly reduce the dust mite population.

There are a number of other measures you can take to monitor dust control:

All carpets should be frequently vacuumed. When buying carpets, choose those of synthetic fibres with low-pile construction. Vacuum all carpets every two to three days.

All dustable surfaces should be gone over two to three times a week, especially in the bedrooms. Make sure that your allergic child is not in the area when you clean.

Wardrobes should be used only for clothes that are worn on a regular basis. Seasonally stored clothes should be kept in a separate area, preferably in a cellar, attic or in dry storage. If seasonal items must be stored in the wardrobe, keep them in garment bags and dust them periodically.

Window shades or washable curtains in the bedrooms are preferable to louvred blinds and heavy drapes.

The dilemma of what to do about a family pet that is known to cause an allergy is difficult to solve. Obviously the answer is to remove the animal as quickly as possible. That's the easy part. But to suddenly give away a beloved animal, 'a relative of my whole family' as one young man described his bulldog to me, is asking a lot of a child. I have come to prefer a step-by-step solution to this nettlesome problem. First banish the dog or cat from the child's section of the house. Then see if the allergy symptoms improve. Sometimes this change alone will be all that's necessary. If step one doesn't bring substantial symptom relief, try restricting the animal to a single room in the house. Then observe the effect. If the previous steps fail, remove the animal from the house entirely, making a home for it in the garage or in an outbuilding. If all else fails, then and then only should you think of finding the animal another home.

Even this last step can have the sting somewhat softened by applying a similar step-by-step approach.

1. Prepare the child in advance, gently explaining why and how the animal will have to be given away. Do not simply snatch the creature up one day and whisk it off without a warning.

2. Find the pet a good home.

3. Make sure the child knows where this home will be, that it will be benevolent, that the pet's new masters will be caring.

4. Be certain the child understands that all this is being done not as a punishment but as a sad and necessary step towards helping the situation.

5. Substitute a nonallergenic pet for the old one. Gerbils, hamsters, guinea pigs and fish are possible replacements.

If your home is heated with a forced-air-type heating system, place filters over the outflow registers. Several layers of cheesecloth make fine homemade filters, though commercial air conditioning filters are more efficient and neat.

A centrally installed humidifier will help control dry-air syndrome. A humidistat can also be used to record relative humidity throughout the house and to determine the efficiency of your humidification unit.

A variety of mechanical devices can be used to filter the air of pollen, dander, dust and smoke fumes, the two basic types being electrostatic precipitators and electronic filters. Although these electronic devices may be of some use in certain cases, allergists are wary of giving a blanket recommendation. Unless scrupulous cleanliness is observed they can end up causing more trouble than they relieve.

IMMUNOTHERAPY

Immunotherapy – or as it is sometimes called, desensitization or hyposensitization – is a method in which a patient is given a regular course of injections containing the allergens to which he or she is clinically allergic. It was very popular, especially for hay fever and house dust mite allergy, until the Committee on Safety of Medicines advised stringent precautions to be observed to make it safe. These restrictions have virtually brought a halt to its use except in the most pressing of circumstances, when it has to be given at a hospital with all its back-up facilities and the patient waiting for two hours after each injection. These precautions were introduced because there had been a number of sudden deaths from anaphylaxis. The makers of at least one brand of desensitizing injection claim there had never been any trouble with their product, so it is always possible that in the future some selectivity may be introduced which would allow some form of desensitization to become a practical proposition again.

It could be very effective where a single allergen had been isolated but in other cases, where testing revealed multiple sensitivities, desensitization was less likely to be successful. The usual practice was to give a course of injections over a period of two to three months before the allergy season and for this to be repeated in three successive years.

COMPLICATIONS THAT MAY OCCUR FROM RHINITIS

Although the symptoms of chronic rhinitis are considered to be primarily annoying, serious complications can develop.

Sinusitis From a developmental point of view there is no general agreement among medical scientists regarding the role of the sinuses. What are they exactly? No one is sure. There are four pairs of sinuses – the maxillary, ethmoid, frontal and sphenoid (see Figure 5, page 148). It has been suggested that these areas are somehow involved with our sense of smell and the production of protective mucus secretions. They also probably play a role in some aspects of voice control and, because they are hollow, their structure reduces the total weight of the head.

The inner surfaces of the sinuses are lined with millions of tiny hairs that regularly propel mucus secretions out of the hollow spaces inside the sinuses, thereby cleaning, lubricating and maintaining these delicate areas in sound working order. Located behind the nose and eyes, sinuses are connected to the nasal passageways by means of tiny openings that allow air to enter and mucus to drain out.

Normally you are not aware of your sinuses until an allergic reaction develops involving the membranes of the nose. At this moment the sinus membranes, which are really a continuation of the nasal membranes, can swell violently and overflow with mucus, blocking the drainage openings leading into the nose. Fluids then become trapped in the passageways, causing a build-up of pressure which eventually can lead to painful, sometimes overpowering headaches. The trapped mucus, meanwhile, becomes an ideal place for viruses and bacteria to set up house, the end result being a sinus infection (sinusitis), which may include chills, fever, dizziness, severe headaches and thick greenish mucus.

Treatment for sinusitis consists of oral decongestants, antihistamines and, when infection is present, antibiotics. Topical nasal preparations in the form of drops or sprays used to shrink the membranes and dry the mucus secretions should not be used for more than five days.

If your child seems to be having discomfort caused by sinus involvement and you are unable to get to the doctor, here are some temporary home remedies.

> Have the child inhale steam from a vaporizer or a pot of boiling water. *Never* leave your child unattended around boiling water or a steam vaporizer. In the twinkling of an eye a scalding can take place.

> The application of a moist heated compress over the sinus areas may help relieve some pain and pressure.

> These remedies are temporary, of course, and should by no means be used to replace adequate medical attention.

In the unusual event of recurring sinus infections that cannot be brought under control with appropriate antibiotic therapy, some form of surgery may be required. In children the most common procedure is called a nasal antrostomy. This operation provides a permanent drainage pathway from the infected sinus into the nose, making it impossible for the mucus to accumulate and become reinfected. This procedure is rarely necessary.

Nosebleeds Any time a child has a problem with chronic nasal symptoms, the possibility of nosebleeds (epistaxis) increases. Children suffering from the irritation of chronic rhinitis will often pick at and bore into their nostrils with a vengeance, despite all pleas and protestations from their parents. Eventually the constant trauma to the delicate nasal membranes causes superficial blood vessels to rupture, especially those on the nasal septum dividing the wall between the nostrils. A bloody nose is the inevitable result.

Nosebleeds tend to occur with increased frequency during the colder months of the year when household heating dries out the nasal linings. All it may take at this point is a minor shock – a strong sneeze, for example – to break the superficial vessels and start the blood flowing. Such nosebleeds are not serious, of course, but they can be irksome to the parents and frightening to the child.

Everyone should know the first aid measures to control a nosebleed. The drill is to get the patient to sit in a chair leaning forward, pinch the soft part of the nose between thumb and index finger, and keep the pressure up for five to ten minutes as measured by the clock. The temptation is to release the pressure too soon. If it does not work the first time, try again for another five to ten minutes; it will often work given long enough. The forward-leaning position is to stop blood being swallowed which may induce vomiting. Blood which collects in the mouth should be spat out. Finally, after the bleeding has stopped, resist all temptation to blow the nose, as this will start it up again! Rarely with children will these measures fail to control the bleeding.

If frequent bleeding continues even after you have increased the humidity level in your home, a visit to an ear, nose and throat specialist may eventually be necessary. More than likely the doctor will solve the problem by applying a chemical or an electric probe to the superficial vessel that has been bleeding. This is a simple, painless procedure that is usually quite effective.

Changes in the dental arch Children who suffer from constant nasal congestion often become chronic mouth breathers. If unchecked, this condition can cause a permanent change in the shape of the mouth that results in the formation of a high-arched palate and changes in the dental arch. Children who are possible candidates for these problems are easily recognized. Perhaps you have seen these children in nursery school or playing in the park. They constantly breathe through their mouths and have persistent nasal congestion or a continually runny nose. The major problem that develops because of the rhinitis is malocclusion of the upper and lower jaws. Unless the chronic nasal problem is treated aggressively, extensive orthodontic work may be required to correct the dental condition.

QUESTIONS AND ANSWERS ABOUT RHINITIS

How severe can hay fever become?

While hay fever is hardly fatal, some children are made so uncomfortable that they become prisoners in their own homes during pollen season. They are less efficient at school, more irritable, and in general quite miserable. Hay-fever symptoms run the gamut from being a mere annoyance to becoming an intransigent, if temporary, agony. Happily, with appropriate medical care almost all children can be helped.

If left untreated, will rhinitis symptoms tend to disappear or will they continue indefinitely?

There are certainly untreated children who, over a period of time, lose their allergic sensitivity and their nasal symptoms. There is no way of knowing whether your child will be among these lucky ones. Very often paediatricians tell parents that their child will outgrow her allergic problem within the next 'several' years and that specific treatment is therefore unnecessary. The reality is that certain children afflicted with allergic rhinitis get better on their own, some get worse, some stay the same. The decision to seek medical advice for a child who has chronic or recurrent rhinitis symptoms should depend on the duration and severity of the complaints.

What will happen if a child's rhinitis condition is allowed to go medically untreated?

At best you will have a very unhappy young person on your hands, and a family that has become utterly frustrated by the child's endless sneezing and complaining. Also, if the symptoms of chronic rhinitis are too long ignored, they might be the forerunner of lower respiratory tract symptoms such as wheezing and difficulty in breathing. This condition does not develop very frequently, contrary to what some doctors may tell parents to scare them into action, but why take the chance?

When parents purchase over-the-counter decongestants or antihistamines, should they ask for these medicines in children's strengths?

Yes. Most antihistamines and decongestants are available in paediatric strengths. The pharmacist or your doctor will give you guidance in this area.

Which forms of medication are preferable for children, nose drops or sprays?

Most children tolerate nasal sprays better than drops. For one thing, decongestant drops are difficult to administer. They almost always 'leak' from the nose into the throat, where their bitter taste quite understandably makes children grimace and complain. A nasal spray is easier to use. The child does not have to lie down – standing is, in fact, the preferred position for taking a spray. Sprays in general deliver a more diffuse application of the medicine over the surface of the nasal membranes. I cannot remind you too often not to allow your child to use a topical nasal decongestant, either in spray form or drops, for more than five days in a row.

DOES ASPIRIN OR PARACETAMOL HELP RHINITIS?

Remember first of all that no aspirin products should be given to children under the age of twelve because of the admittedly very rare but potentially fatal Reye's syndrome.

Neither of these analgesics by themselves helps rhinitis. If a headache happens to accompany a rhinitis attack, as it occasionally does, an analgesic will probably help relieve it. It will not reduce the primary symptoms of the rhinitis alone.

Why do some allergic children develop dark circles under their eyes?

These dark circles are popularly known as 'allergic shiners'. They are not due to lack of sleep or poor eating habits but are produced by the slow movement of blood, which collects in the capillary beds under the eyes. The blood flow is slowed by the allergic swelling that occurs in the nasal mucous membranes. The darkness itself is due to a 'pooling' of venous blood that accumulates in these thin-walled superficial blood vessels under the eyes. During the times of year when a child has allergic symptoms, he may develop these shiners on a fairly regularly basis. They have no sinister significance. When the season passes and swelling in the nose recedes, they will disappear. Allergic shiners are nothing to be alarmed about and in no way indicate any underlying pathology, except for the allergic condition.

At what age can the symptoms of allergic rhinitis begin?

In theory, rhinitis can start at any age. The youngest rhinitis patient I can recall was a five-day-old infant named David who was allergic to his formula and developed severe nasal obstruction. When a nonmilk formula was introduced into David's diet, his nasal symptoms disappeared. In practice this case is quite unusual because of the exceptionally early onset of symptoms. Typically, seasonal allergic symptoms appear only after a child has become sensitized to aero-allergens such as trees, grass or weed pollens, a process of exposure that ordinarily takes several years before symptoms become apparent.

What part, if any, do stress and emotional anxiety play in the development of rhinitis?

In my opinion the development of *allergic* rhinitis is not influenced by emotional factors. Some forms of chronic rhinitis, specifically vasomotor rhinitis, can and quite often will be aggravated by periods of stress and anxiety.

Are there particular times of day when a child's rhinitis becomes better or worse?

Seasonal rhinitis sufferers generally have their most intense symptoms in the early morning and in the late afternoon or early evening. These are the times of day when plants usually release their pollen into the air.

Can houseplants cause allergic rhinitis?

Rarely. The only potential problem may be found in the soil. Occasionally, moulds that thrive in potting soil can irritate the allergies of highly mould-sensitive children. On the whole, for the majority of children nonflowering houseplants are nothing to worry about.

Teachers will sometimes insist that a child suffering from chronic rhinitis actually has a cold and should be kept out of school. How should parents deal with such a situation?

If a child is diagnosed as having an allergic problem, either of a seasonal or year-round nature, the doctor should provide you with a note to this effect; the note should then be sent on to the proper school authorities. The real difficulty comes at those times when the child develops a cold *superimposed* on an underlying allergic condition and it becomes difficult to tell the two apart. In such situations there are still certain criteria that can be applied:

If the child has a fever, she should be kept home.

If mucus coming from the child's nose is thick and yellowish, an infection is most likely the cause of the symptoms, not an allergy.

If the child complains of symptoms such as aches and pains, a viral infection may be present.

CHAPTER SEVEN

Hives and Angioedema

HIVES (URTICARIA)

Anyone who has ever been plagued by hives or who has stood helplessly by and watched a family member suffer the relentless itching (pruritis) this ailment brings will agree that hives can literally drive a person mad. Some of the most uncomfortable and troubled patients I have seen over the past twenty years have been victims of this most unpleasant condition.

Appearing on the surface of the skin as well-outlined raised areas, hives tend to have a whitish or reddish coloration. There is no typical size for the lesions themselves; they can be as small as a pencil eraser or large enough to cover an entire arm or leg. Similarly, there is no specific part of the body more prone to hives than any other; we are susceptible from the tops of our heads to the soles of our feet, and it is even possible to develop lesions internally along the length of the intestinal tract. An attack of hives can consist of one large hive, several hives located in different parts of the body, or a cluster of many small hives concentrated in a specific area. Sometimes individual welts will 'grow together', forming a single large, irregularly shaped swelling which covers a large section of the body. Lesions of this size are known as giant hives.

The itching sensation associated with hives is the most disheartening part of it all. I have seen infants practically tear their skin off in a futile attempt to find relief. The localized itching and swelling of hives is caused by the leakage of fluids from the smallest blood vessels just beneath the surface of the skin after histamine is released during an allergic reaction.

As a rule, an eruption of hives appears without warning, makes the child intensely uncomfortable for several hours, then slowly subsides. Occasionally, though, hives may be present for considerably longer, sometimes for months or even years. Technically speaking, hives that recur for six weeks or more are defined as chronic, six weeks or less, acute. The chance of determining the actual cause of acute hives is less than 30 per cent. Fortunately in both situations, while the origin is difficult to determine, medical relief of symptoms is usually within reach.

It is estimated that 10 to 20 per cent of the population will at one time or another suffer from an episode of hives. Acute urticaria tends to appear more frequently among people who are allergic; chronic hives strikes the allergic and nonallergic child with equal frequency.

ANGIOEDEMA

Simply stated, angioedema represents a hive that has invaded the deeper skin layers. The swelling of angioedema is usually more spread out and less distinct. A big difference between hives and angioedema is that the first itches and the second doesn't. The persistent itching so closely associated with hives occurs because the nerves transmitting the 'itch sensation' are located in the outermost skin layers where the hives develop. Angioedema, on the other hand, rarely produces itching, as the superficial free nerve endings are not affected. Indeed, it is the extreme swelling associated with angioedema that may occasionally cause pain rather than itching, especially if the swelling occurs in areas of the body where the skin is tightly stretched, such as on the fingers.

While hives can certainly drive you to distraction they are rarely, if ever, the cause of a potentially life-threatening situation. Angioedema, on the other hand, if it involves areas such as the tongue, mouth or windpipe (trachea), may prove fatal if it continues without appropriate medical attention.

THE PHYSIOLOGY OF HIVES

Hives develop when the chemical mediator histamine is secreted into the bloodstream and body tissues. This substance can be released by several different mechanisms, the most common being an allergic reaction. Regardless of the triggering factor, the end result of histamine in the superficial skin layers is the same: leakage of fluid out of the small blood vessels, localized swelling, the consequent production of wheals, and the all-too-familiar sensation of unrelenting itching. (For a detailed description of the mechanism of histamine release and the part it plays in the allergic process, see page 21.)

Mysteries remain, of course, as to how this entire process works. To date, researchers have been unable to prove that histamine is the only mediator involved in hive formation; there may well be others we have not yet discovered. The question of why certain children develop allergic responses while others do not remains one of the enduring riddles in allergy research.

HELPING YOUR DOCTOR DIAGNOSE THE CAUSE OF HIVES

Hives and angioedema are usually easy to identify; discovering the causes behind them is far more difficult. You can help by becoming a careful observer and by keeping a watchful eye out for answers to the following pertinent questions, many of which you will be asked at the time of your child's first medical consultation:

When do the hives appear?

On which parts of the body are they located?

How long do they last? Do they tend to come and go or do they remain for prolonged periods of time?

Describe their size and appearance.

How frequently do they occur? What are the average time intervals between attacks?

Under what particular circumstances, if any, do they seem to occur?

Are any unusual circumstances present when the rash appears?

What foods has the child eaten in the twenty-four-hour period preceding the onset? (Be alert for new or unusual foods that have recently been introduced, especially those that classically cause allergic responses – chocolate, eggs, citrus fruits, shellfish, strawberries, wheat, nuts and milk.)

Has there been recent exposure at school or at home to unusual substances: chemicals, pesticides, hobby paints and glues, industrial materials?

Has the child recently experienced added emotional stress owing to conflicts with friends, family, school situations, general life circumstances? Do the hives tend to appear after periods of excitement or temper tantrums?

What is the current state of the child's overall health? Is he convalescing from any long-term ailment?

Do other symptoms ever accompany the hives? If so, describe them.

Has the child recently received an inoculation of any kind?

Has the child recently started a course of new drugs, nose drops, sprays, tonics, laxatives, vitamins, cold tablets or other medication?

Has the child had any recent problems related to teeth, the intestinal tract, the urinary tract, fungal infections, appendicitis or tonsils?

Have you recently made any changes in your household cleaning or personal products such as soaps, detergents, bleaches and fabric softeners, shampoos, cosmetics, hair sprays, bath powders, dyes, mouthwashes, nail polish, toothpaste, and so on?

Have you recently brought any new or unusual items into the house such as furniture, curtains, chemicals? Have you painted your house lately?

Does the child tend to develop hives after touching cold objects such as snow or ice cubes?

Do hot or cold showers affect the child's condition?

Does any particular type of insect infest your home or immediate environment? Does the child experience allergic reactions to any type of insect bite?

Do the hives appear after a period of physical exertion and exercise?

Have you recently brought a pet into the house? Are there animals of any kind in the home environment? What are they?

Have you and/or the child recently visited new places? Have you recently moved?

This list represents only a partial sampling of the questions an allergist might ask during an initial evaluation session *and* which you as parent should be prepared, as best you can, to answer thoroughly. The point must be made again that your doctor, even armed with answers to all the questions he may ask, can diagnose the cause of acute hives only in *less* than 30 per cent of cases, while the cause of chronic hives can be diagnosed in less than *10* to *20* per cent. Not very happy statistics. But before you close this book and walk away, you should know that even if the cause of the hives ultimately eludes everyone, parents, doctor and patient alike, the chances of medically *controlling* them remain very, very good.

FACTORS THAT TRIGGER HIVES

If I tried to write down all the possible causes of hives, hundreds of pages would soon be filled with lists of foods, chemical agents, medical conditions, insects, and virtually every kind of pharmacological agent in use today. The subject is vastly complex and extremely confusing. Still, an attempt must be made. The sections that follow, though certainly not inclusive of all the substances and situations that may cause hives, is complete enough to give you some idea of what to stay away from as well as where the major points of danger lie.

Drugs Hives can develop owing to an allergic drug reaction or drug intolerance (see pages 228 and 232). Medicines that can cause such trouble include:

> any antibiotics
>
> aspirin
>
> barbiturates
>
> codeine
>
> insulin
>
> iodides
>
> penicillin
>
> sulpha drugs
>
> tetanus antitoxin (horse serum)

Drugs of any type can cause hives. Discuss all medications with your doctor to decide if you should continue to use them or if there are substitutes. In the paediatric population, penicillin and its derivatives are probably the most likely of all drugs to trigger acute hives. Aspirin, of course, should not be given to children under twelve, but it is a well-known cause of hives. Paracetamol is a more suitable mild analgesic, either in its generic form, which is the cheapest and just as effective, or under the various brand names which are possibly more palatable.

A similar negative reaction may be caused by azo dyes, especially tartrazine. This chemical dye can be yellow, red or purple and is used in foods and in many medicinal drugs including antihistamines. Another common preservative, benzoic acid, is present in many foods and drugs and can cause hives. The list of possible hive-producing substances by no means stops here and includes just about *any* drug or chemical.

It is therefore vitally important that parents keep an accurate record of all medications taken by their child, both prescription and over-the-counter varieties. This is one area of the child's personal medical history an allergist will most likely spend a good deal of time discussing with you.

Infection The possible cause-and-effect relationship between chronic low-grade infections of the tonsils, adenoids, sinuses, teeth, gall bladder or urinary tract and the development of hives has been debated by allergists for many years, and the final answer has yet to be resolved. I myself recall having seen two or three chronic hive sufferers whose symptoms disappeared when an unsuspected infection was discovered and treated. While I can provide no clear-cut medical reason why infection should be capable of causing hives I do believe that for a very small number of patients such a relationship exists. Cases of this sort, I would add, are extremely rare and would certainly account for only a tiny percentage of urticarial episodes.

Infestation with parasites Parasitic infection is another possible but somewhat unusual cause of chronic hives. The presence of animals in the home, poor personal hygiene habits, or recent trips taken to exotic places are all subjects your allergist will probably bring up with you at the initial interview. It is not easy to detect the presence of parasites in a person's body under any circumstances, and repeated examinations of multiple fresh stool specimens may be necessary if parasites are suspected. Once a specific type of parasite has been found, appropriate treatment is available.

Foods and food additives Though it is not possible to collect accurate statistics on the number of children who actually suffer from food-related hives, we know that foods are a common cause. Hives can be triggered either by the foods themselves or by the chemical additives in them. Several of the more common offending foods include dairy products, eggs, nuts (including peanuts), citrus fruits, tomatoes and shellfish. To this list add the multitudinous number of chemical additives, now somewhere in the hundreds, used in the growing, freshening and preserving of the foods we consume every day. Some of the more important representatives of this group include the tartrazine food dyes and preservatives such as sodium benzoate, sulphite or metabisulphite. Soy products, which have been used as substitutes for milk-based infant formulas, can also trigger hives. With the increased use of soy products in our diet, allergists have been discovering more people who are allergic to this food.

Three important points to note about food-induced hives:

Acute urticaria is likely to be triggered by seasonal or unusual foods such as fresh vegetables and fruit, shellfish or strawberries.

Chronic urticaria is likely to be triggered by foods which are part of the normal daily diet such as wheat, milk or eggs.

Although an outbreak of hives usually follows immediately after the offending foods have been eaten, occasionally as much as eighteen to twenty-four hours may elapse before the first lesions appear.

What should you do? While it is, of course, not always possible to pinpoint which ingested substances are responsible for hives, the use of a food diary will help. In this written record, *all* the foods your child eats each day must be carefully recorded. The list should cover snacks, school lunches, and 'extracurricular' eating of any kind, including forbidden sweets. Also useful is an elimination diet in which specific foods and food groups are removed from the child's menu and any reaction to this change of diet is observed and recorded. As an example, if you suspect that your child's hives are triggered by milk, you can eliminate *all* dairy products from her diet for seven to ten days, noting how much, if at all, the hives have improved. There is a further discussion of foods and food allergies in general in the chapter on food allergies. There is also a listing of foods that may cause hives starting on page 213.

Insect stings and bites Before you can become allergic to a specific insect, you must be stung at least once by this creature in order to become sensitized. Though insect-induced hives are most often triggered by attacks from members of the order *Hymenoptera* – bees, wasps and hornets – several other flying and crawling creatures can be responsible.

Papular urticaria, a hivelike eruption found primarily on the lower extremities, is caused by bites from bedbugs, fleas and mites. These lesions are usually more persistent than typical hives, smaller in appearance, and quite itchy.

In a child who has been sensitized to a specific caterpillar, contact with the wiggly creature will cause a linear-appearing itchy skin rash to develop. In Britain the caterpillars of the brown-tail and yellow-tail moths are especially likely to cause this problem; the rash is known as caterpillar dermatitis. Children who touch these caterpillars should immediately wash those parts of their bodies that have been in contact with the creatures.

Occasionally, fly and mosquito stings can trigger hives. For further specifics on insect sting reactions, see the following chapter.

Inhalants Occasionally reports are heard in an allergist's consulting room of hives being triggered by inhalants such as dander or pollen. If such a relationship can be firmly documented, immunotherapy may be one method of helping the situation. From my experience, inhalant-caused hives are extremely unusual.

Physical agents A wide variety of physical agents and conditions can produce an urticarial response. The following are the most common.

Sometimes called skin writing, *dermatographism* is an acute sensitivity of the skin to the force of friction. One of the most common types of physical urticaria, it takes the form of hivelike lesions that appear over any area that has recently been scraped or rubbed. The response can easily be elicited in sensitive children by running the blunt tip of a pen or pencil along the arms or legs; in a relatively short time a raised, reddened, occasionally itchy linear eruption will appear where the skin was stroked.

For some children, it also turns out, dermatographism can be a source of enormous pride and delight. Such youngsters have a great deal of fun allowing friends to draw pictures on their legs or to play noughts and crosses across their forearms, making them the centre of envy and attention. Perhaps this transformation of a liability into an asset is a blessing for the child too, for dermatographism is a permanent, lifetime phenomenon – nothing more, really, than a manifestation of highly sensitive skin.

Hives caused by *sudden exposure to low temperatures* (cold urticaria) – e.g. running into the ocean, going from a warm house into the cold winter air – can be a potentially serious problem, triggering unpleasant symptoms such as headache, wheezing and on rare occasions severe breathing difficulties. A fifteen-year-old patient of mine named Jim once went for a swim in an icy mountain pond. Almost from the moment he entered the water his skin began to break out in hives from head to foot, and within a few minutes his breathing had become laboured. Fortunately, there was a hospital ten minutes away, and after an injection of adrenaline Jim's rash and wheezing subsided. Such a reaction is rare, it must be pointed out, and usually symptoms remain local, i.e., hives develop on the face and ungloved hands of a person taking a walk on a cold, windy day; an itchy rash appears on the hands when handling an ice cube. Typically, the symptoms of cold urticaria develop after exposure to the cold has taken place and the body is beginning to warm up. Jim's situation is somewhat unusual; however, it certainly is potentially dangerous for anyone who has this condition to jump into the sea or dive into a pool!

The intensity of the symptoms that develop after exposure to a cold challenge will depend on the size of the body area chilled. For example, whenever Jane goes for a walk on a cold, wintry day, hives appear only on her face and hands (if she is not wearing gloves). Jim, on the other hand, rapidly developed generalized hives and breathing difficulties when his entire body was submerged into the pool. In either case there is no completely effective treatment, though the following measures may be taken to lessen the symptoms.

During the cold months of the year, cover the child's body as fully as possible whenever he ventures outdoors. This means gloves, hats, scarves, the works.

In the summertime, make sure the child enters the sea or swimming pool s-l-o-w-l-y. Diving is, of course, out of the question, as are any of the sudden-immersion methods (such as pushing) that children and teenagers so enjoy. Let the child get acclimatized to the water gradually, by degrees, especially when about to enter deep or potentially dangerous areas such as those found in a lake or the sea.

The antihistamine Periactin (cyproheptadine) is usually effective in blocking the effects of cold urticaria. It is useful, however, only when administered *before* exposure.

If you suspect that your child is suffering from cold urticaria, test your hunch by performing the 'ice-cube test'. Place an ice cube directly on the child's forearm. Leave it there for five minutes, then take it away and examine the contact area. If, as the area rewarms, a red, raised, itchy wheal appears on the spot in the exact shape of the ice cube, this is a positive response. This proves that cold urticaria is present.

Another form of urticaria is called *cholinergic urticaria*. This condition develops as a response to emotional stress, vigorous physical exertion, or heat exposure. The rash consists of many very small (less than one-eighth-inch) raised wheals which are all intensely itchy.

Still another temperature-related rash is so-called *localized heat urticaria*. As its name suggests, it takes place on skin surfaces that are locally heated by a sun lamp, a flame, whatever. Relatively few cases have ever been recorded of this disorder, and I personally have never seen one.

In certain susceptible people, sunlight has the potential of producing a localized skin response called *solar urticaria*. This rash appears as hives on areas of the body frequently and directly exposed to the sun. Usually seen in tropical or desert climates, it is by no means geographically limited and is occasionally reported in colder regions, especially during the summer months. Solar urticaria is relatively unusual.

An unusual form of hives called *vibratory angioedema* is produced by skin contact with a rapidly shaking object, especially a mechanical object such as a throttle or the handle of a running lawn mower. The condition is rare and invariably inherited. Symptoms consist of hives, redness and localized swelling of the skin following stimulation of the contact area. The condition is usually noticed early in childhood and tends to persist throughout life. While it is rarely cause for serious concern, there is no specific cure for vibratory angioedema other than avoidance of contact with vibratory stimuli.

Typically *pressure urticaria and angioedema* results from a response, usually delayed, to persistent pressure applied to various parts of the body. Tight clothing, belts, boots, bra straps, elastic on socks, a tight grip on a tennis racket, sitting in the same position for hours, any prolonged pressure can provoke it. Its identifying rash consists of itchy deep red wheals which appear up to four to six hours after the pressure stimulation has ceased.

Another unusual form of hives, *aquagenic urticaria*, is produced by skin contact with hot or cold water. Its characteristic rash has the same appearance as that caused by cholinergic urticaria, which is identified by its extremely small, red, extraordinarily itchy wheals. Very little is understood about this condition at present. As far as we know, it involves only a tiny percentage of people who develop hives.

In *exercise-induced urticaria*, hives or angioedema appear after a period of strenuous physical activity. While such outbreaks are usually mild, a particularly severe form does exist called exercise-induced anaphylaxis. I witnessed one such case several years ago. A teenage jogger taking his daily run suddenly developed severe wheezing along with an outbreak of hives. Gripped with an agonizing inability to catch his breath, the boy had to be rushed to a hospital where emergency measures with oxygen and adrenaline revived him. As with several of the other unusual varieties of urticaria mentioned, this condition is extremely rare.

Miscellaneous causes of hives A number of common and unusual urticarial conditions exist that do not fit into any of the categories mentioned so far.

Urticaria pigmentosa is a rather uncommon condition which consists of localized, slightly raised pigmented lesions. These areas are collections of mast cells under the skin. (Mast cells, you will recall, are white blood cells containing large amounts of histamine, the primary cause of hive formation.) If these areas are stroked or rubbed, histamine will be released from the cells and local hive formation will occur. Urticaria pigmentosa generally appears during the early childhood years and quite often vanishes when a youngster reaches puberty.

Hives may also appear as symptoms of other diseases Ailments involving the collagen-vascular system (the connective and blood vessel systems) may produce chronic hives as early symptoms of an underlying condition. In fact, chronic generalized urticaria may on a rare occasion be an early symptom of a systemic disease such as rheumatoid arthritis, systemic lupus erythematosis, endocrine problems (especially hyperthyroidism), Hodgkin's disease or cancer of the colon. The point must be stressed, however, that these cases are extremely unusual; I have never seen a case in this category.

While anxiety-producing problems with family, friends, school, and so on can sometimes aggravate an existing urticarial condition, hives occurring *solely* on the basis of emotional problems are not very common. Let me also add that when a child's personal history is taken at the allergist's consulting room, questions regarding the relationship between hives and the child's emotional state will inevitably be asked. Family members should be on guard against holding back critical information in this area out of fear of appearing inadequate or from worry about putting their child in a bad light. Remember, the doctor's interest is not in judging you or your child, only in eliminating the symptoms.

Hereditary angioedema (HAE) is caused by the absence or improper functioning of a specific enzyme of the complement system (known technically as Cl-esterase inhibitor) and is clinically characterized by recurring attacks of painful angioedema typically involving the skin and mucous membranes of the upper respiratory system and gastrointestinal tracts. These attacks in some patients may be triggered by mild physical trauma such as bumping into a wall or door. If your child has repeated complaints of abdominal pain and suffers from frequent swelling of the face and extremities, these symptoms should make you suspicious enough to contact your doctor. The condition can be diagnosed by means of specific blood tests. Hereditary angioedema is not a disease to be taken lightly. When swelling involves the upper airways, the larynx can become blocked; death from suffocation has been reported in approximately 10 to 20 per cent of HAE patients. Fortunately, laryngeal swelling usually takes several hours to develop, so that when and if respiratory involvement is discovered, HAE sufferers can usually get themselves to a doctor or a hospital before the attack becomes too severe. Hereditary angioedema, rare as it is, can definitely be *a life-threatening disease* and should be kept under strict medical supervision. Specific drug therapy is available today to control the condition.

A diagnosis of *idiopathic urticaria*, or idiopathic angioedema, is the medical way of saying that we simply do not know what specific factors are causing the problem. This is the ultimate diagnosis in 50 to 70 per cent of acute urticarial cases and 80 to 90 per cent of chronic urticaria and angioedema cases.

DIAGNOSTIC TESTING FOR HIVES

In theory there is no limit to the number of diagnostic tests that can be ordered for a child with hives. In addition to blood samples, stool examinations and X-ray studies, consultations with a wide variety of specialists may be recommended. I do not advocate this zealous approach. I feel that after obtaining a detailed personal history and performing a thorough physical examination, a few basic screening tests are all that is needed to make a preliminary diagnosis and suggest a course of treatment. The first laboratory tests I generally order include:

A full blood count (FBC) (see page 36)

a urinalysis

an erythrocyte sedimentation rate determination test, used as a general screening test for infection or inflammation in the body.

If information is revealed in the child's personal history that suggests a specific cause for her hives, a number of other tests may possibly be ordered to confirm or disprove these suspicions. Such tests run the gamut from highly specific enzyme analysis to challenge tests using particular foods or other allergens. Your doctor will suggest the tests which are most appropriate.

When the laboratory evaluation has been completed, and if the tests fail to show anything unusual, a diagnosis of idiopathic urticaria, either acute or chronic, will then be justified. Attention must next be focused on treatment.

TREATMENT OF HIVES AND ANGIOEDEMA

ENVIRONMENTAL CONTROL AND ELIMINATION PROCEDURES

It is obvious that if the underlying cause of hives can be identified – foods, animals, chemicals, medicines or whatever – removal of these substances from the patient's environment will usually cure the condition. While it is not always easy to determine the cause of hives, once the discovery has been made avoidance is the best way to clear it up.

A few general recommendations can be made:

Do not give your child any aspirin-containing preparations; use paracetamol as a substitute.

Read food labels carefully and keep away from preservatives such as benzoates and members of the sulphite family. Do not use foods or medicines containing tartrazine dyes, especially E102.

If a pet dog or cat has proved to be the culprit causing the hives, then contact with the animal must be avoided.

For some of the more unusual types of physical stimuli (hot, cold, pressure, exertion) that may trigger the hives, the obvious recommendation is to avoid the situation that may bring on the symptoms.

USEFUL MEDICATION FOR HIVES

Antihistamines These drugs represent the first line of defence against symptoms of recurring urticaria; for the majority of patients, one or a combination of antihistamines will often be all the medication needed. As is commonly the case with antihistamines, however, it may take several tries on the doctor's part before the most effective antihistamine is discovered. While there are many antihistamines to choose from, it has been my clinical experience that hydroxyzine, marketed as Atarax, is the most effective for hives. I gradually increase the dose of this drug until the hives have disappeared completely for seven to ten days and then slowly lower the dose over a two-to-four week period. At the end of this time the hives have usually disappeared, and in approximately 80 to 90 per cent of cases they do not return. Other antihistamines such as diphenhydramine (marketed as Benadryl) and cyproheptadine (marketed as Periactin) may be substituted for hydroxyzine if it cannot be tolerated or if it does not work. (For detailed information on antihistamines, see the chapter on asthma.)

Adrenaline For sudden episodes of severe, generalized hives or angioedema, treatment with adrenaline by injection usually brings rapid relief, though of a relatively short duration.

Orciprenalol and Terbutaline Orciprenalol, marketed as Alupent, and terbutaline, marketed as Bricanyl, are occasionally prescribed for hives in combination with an antihistamine. Such combinations are sometimes more effective than the antihistamine alone.

Corticosteroids Corticosteroids, when given in an appropriate dose, will successfully control almost all difficult cases of hives and angioedema. Because of their potentially dangerous side effects, however, these powerful preparations should be reserved for instances in which all other medications prove ineffective.

Regarding the dose, enough steroid medication should be given to suppress the hives. The duration of treatment should be the shortest possible time necessary to bring the symptoms under control. When the patient has been free of hives for three to four days, the dose can be decreased over the next four to six days. If steroids are abruptly discontinued, sometimes the hives will rebound in a more severe form; this is the reason for tapering the dose.

LAST THOUGHTS

The ultimate outcome of urticaria and angioedema treatment depends on the underlying cause. Most acute cases are mild and self-limited; they appear and vanish without causing much difficulty. Soothing lotions such as calamine help in these situations, as do applications of wet baking soda or oatmeal. Avoid, however, Caladryl, a calamine lotion containing Benadryl that is often used to provide symptomatic relief for patients with hives. Benadryl alone is an excellent antihistamine when taken by mouth, but when used topically it can sensitize the skin and may cause a contact dermatitis. Anyone suffering from hives certainly doesn't need a second skin condition to worry about! Often nothing more elaborate than an over-the-counter cortisone ointment will do the trick. Whatever physical causes are the underlying trigger of this disorder, avoidance of the offending stimuli should control the symptoms. On the other hand, if urticaria is due to an underlying systemic disease, the outcome will naturally depend on the nature of the disease and the effectiveness of its treatment.

Finally, parents should be aware that chronic urticaria has a highly variable course: the symptoms may be present for several months or for many years. Periodic recurrences are not uncommon, though they are by no means guaranteed. In most cases this ailment is highly exasperating, at times causing itching so intense that patients feel like jumping out of their skins. Fortunately, except when associated with hereditary angioedema or with a malignant disease, urticaria is rarely life-threatening and can usually be kept well controlled.

QUESTIONS AND ANSWERS ON HIVES AND ANGIOEDEMA

Should I be concerned if my child gets an occasional hive?

The appearance of one or two hives now and then is nothing to worry about. If the lesions are present for a short while and then clear up without medication, I would certainly not recommend consulting a professional. If, however, the hives are numerous, if they return frequently, and if they last for more than a day or so at a time, it would then be appropriate to discuss the situation with a doctor.

Can hives be contagious?

The answer is a very definite no. You cannot 'catch' hives by being in contact with someone who has them, just as you cannot catch asthma, angioedema and most other allergic ailments.

Are allergy injections appropriate for the treatment of hives?

It is theoretically possible for a child to develop hives as a result of a seasonal pollen sensitivity. In such an instance an argument could be made for the use of immunotherapy. Let me add, however, that in my many years of practice I have never seen such a case.

What role, if any, does climate or seasonal change play in chronic urticaria?

For most urticaria sufferers the changing seasons and variations in daily climate play little or no role in their conditions. For those few children whose hives are triggered by winter weather (cold urticaria) or exposure to the sun (solar urticaria), a relationship obviously exists between the ailment and the season of the year. For these children appropriate precautions are always in order – wearing gloves and scarves in cold weather, using sun screens out of doors.

CHAPTER EIGHT

Insect Sting Allergies

Andy, an active, outgoing six-year-old, was in the school playground one day during break. Picking up a rock, he felt a sharp stinging sensation in his right hand. Quickly turning pale and becoming very anxious, he was taken to the school nurse, who cleaned what had become a large swelling on his wrist. Within a few minutes Andy seemed to be comfortable and was sent back to class. Five minutes later he returned to the sickroom, complaining this time of chest pains; he was again very pale and quite uneasy. The school contacted his mother and she called the family doctor. By this time Andy was clearly in severe discomfort and an ambulance was called to transport him to the local hospital.

In the hospital, Andy was treated for what appeared to be a generalized reaction to an insect sting. Within an hour he was fine and ready to be discharged. The doctor's initial impression was that Andy had not reacted allergically to the sting but had experienced a fright response from the pain. The child was referred to me to answer a number of his parents' questions. Was Andy really allergic to insect stings, and if so, what could be done about it? What medicines should the family keep at home and in school to cope with the problem? What would happen if Andy was stung again? Could such a reaction be triggered by fear alone? Could such a sting be fatal?

These are only some of the many questions asked thousands of times each year by parents of children who are allergic to insect stings. I want to review with you the current state of our knowledge regarding this frightening and often misunderstood condition, and then I will tell you how to cope with this situation.

The first fatality formally attributed to a wasp sting occurred in Egypt in 2641 B.C. The illustrious victim, according to temple hieroglyphics, was none other than the pharaoh himself, a ruler named Menes. Throughout unrecorded and recorded history stinging insects have regularly plagued humanity, though no one knows exactly how many of us are actually attacked each year by members of the more dangerous varieties, especially the *Hymenoptera* order of insects, whose ranks include bees, wasps, hornets and the 'fire ant'. The multitude of people annually attacked by these aggressive creatures is in the millions, of course, but, happily, estimates from studies suggest that 99.5 per cent of victims have nothing more serious to worry about than a little temporary discomfort.

For our purposes there remains the one-half of 1 per cent to consider, and for these people the situation may be hazardous and even life-threatening – on average four reported deaths each year are *directly* attributed to insect sting reactions. Fortunately for young people, the vast majority of these fatalities occur in adults, and in fact it is very unusual for a child to die from a sting of any kind, even if the child is highly allergic. Still, caution is the watchword, especially if you know for certain that your child is vulnerable. First, let's identify the cast of villains.

THE ORDER HYMENOPTERA

Within this biological group the female alone is capable of delivering a sting. We know this for certain because only the female possesses a stinger. Important among the *Hymenoptera* are the following families of insects:

Apidae The principal here is the honeybee (see Figure 6), a small, hairy insect decorated with yellow or tan stripes. Honeybees live in man-made hives or in hives constructed in trees, stumps and caves. As a rule, honeybees are relatively unaggressive creatures; most stings occur when bees are stepped on or when their hives are menaced.

Unfortunately for the bee, its stinger and its intestines are attached to one another. Since the bee inevitably eviscerates itself when trying to pull its barbed stinger free from the sting site, the delivery of its sting is tantamount to suicide. (Honeybees are the only members of the order *Hymenoptera* with barbed stingers.)

Thus a child can be stung only once by the same bee, and anyone who shows signs of several bee stings has, *ipso facto*, been stung by several different attackers. Another point: if your child has been stung and the stinger is visible and protruding, remember that significant amounts of venom are still present in the sac attached to it. Grabbing the stinger as if it were a splinter and moving it around will only end up forcing more venom into the unfortunate victim. The best thing to do under these circumstances is to flick the stinger off with the thumb and forefinger, as quickly and as smoothly as possible.

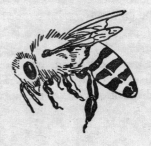
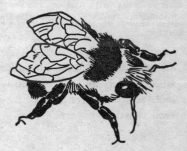

Figure 6   Honeybee   Figure 7   Bumblebee

Bombidae The most important member in this group is the bumblebee (see Figure 7). This large, noisy, ponderous creature covered with yellow and black bands is almost never guilty of stinging anyone. It does have the necessary apparatus to sting, but it takes enormous aggressiveness on the part of any adult or child to force an attack. In general, despite their frightening appearance, bumblebees are not insects to worry about.

Vespidae Wasps. These creatures have a narrow hairless body characterized by a tapered waist (see Figure 8(b)). Wasps build their small open honeycombed nests in trees, shrubs and especially in the eaves of houses. They can deliver a painful sting when riled. Hornets (see Figure 8(a)) can be very aggressive, but they are uncommon. Their sting can be very painful. They have

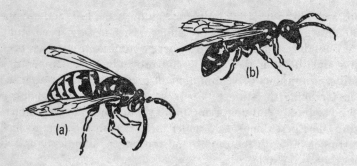

Figure 8(a) Hornet and (b) Wasp

an unbarbed stinger. This means the insect can sting, remove its stinger safely and sting again without suffering any ill effects. This fact, added to its nervous, irascible disposition, makes the hornet well worth avoiding.

CLINICAL REACTIONS TO INSECT STINGS

What reactions might you expect following the sting of a member of the *Hymenoptera* order? In general, there are three types: local, generalized multi-organ system response, and unusual.

Local reactions A local reaction is the type of response a *non*allergic individual develops when stung. It consists of a sharp, burning sensation at the site of the sting, caused by toxic substances contained in the insect's venom. Within five to fifteen minutes local swelling and redness will appear, and all signs of the reaction usually vanish within twelve to twenty-four hours. At times a local reaction can also involve a large area of the body: a hand, an arm or even the whole face. The important thing to remember when such a thing occurs is that this response, no matter how dramatic and uncomfortable it may be, is in no way life-threatening.

Generalized multi-organ system response If a child is stung on the arm, and if hives and breathing difficulties soon develop, that child is experiencing what is known as an anaphylactic reaction. The crucial thing to observe is whether or not the developing symptoms involve areas of the body distant from the sting site. If that is the situation, you can be certain that an allergic response is taking place. A generalized or constitutional reaction requires *prompt medical treatment*. Remember, if your child is stung on the finger and her face becomes swollen – get to a doctor!

Observe also that a generalized reaction, or for that matter any kind of allergic response to an insect sting, can occur *only* after a person has been sensitized to the venom of that insect. In other words, to develop an allergic sensitivity to an insect your child must have been stung by the same creature or a related family member at least once and possibly many times at some earlier date. The intensity of the response that follows can range from a mild outbreak of hives to a severe systemic reaction causing a sudden drop in blood pressure, generalized swelling, a tight sensation in the throat, and difficulty in breathing. Death can ultimately result if the condition is not treated promptly.

Allergic reactions can begin within minutes after the sting or several hours after the attack. The symptoms can be mild, characterized by skin eruptions, general redness and itching, hives and angioedema (swelling of the lips, nose and ears). Or they may be far more serious, consisting of some or all of the following:

> involvement of the airways. Symptoms may include tightness in the chest, shortness of breath, hoarse voice (which comes from swelling of the larynx and throat) and wheezing

> a severe drop in blood pressure (hypotension) with accompanying confusion, paleness and possible loss of consciousness.

> intestinal symptoms such as nausea, vomiting and pain

In its most severe form an anaphylactic reaction to a sting can be fatal. As mentioned earlier, however, it is extremely rare for children to die from such causes.

Generalized toxic reactions are produced not by an allergy

but by a reaction to the poisonous substances in the insect's venom. This type of reaction occurs only after someone has received many, many stings within a short period of time. The accumulated toxins contained in the venom are thought to be responsible for the following symptoms:

headache

dizziness

fever

gastrointestinal complaints: nausea, vomiting, pain, diarrhoea

convulsions

Unusual or atypical reactions These reactions, not caused by an allergic condition, are almost always delayed in their onset. The parts of the body involved are almost always the vascular and nervous systems. Responses include clotting defects in the blood, bloody diarrhoea, neuritis and partial paralysis. Less common are fever, joint aches and pains, enlargement and tenderness of the lymph nodes, hives and angioedema. When these somewhat mysterious symptoms do occur, they may last only a day or so, or they may continue for several weeks. In general, these reactions are quite rare.

DIAGNOSING ALLERGIC INSECT STING REACTIONS

How does your doctor go about determining whether or not your child has actually had an allergic sting reaction? There are several ways.

As I have stressed in preceding chapters, the more complete the presentation of the child's personal medical history at the time of the initial consultation, the easier it will be for an allergist to piece together the evidence and make a specific diagnosis. This rule holds particularly true for insect stings. Why? Referral to an allergist for an insect sensitivity usually takes place days to weeks after the reaction to the sting has subsided. A physical examination will be given, of course, but since the symptoms have disappeared there is not a lot to be learned from this avenue of investigation. The personal history therefore emerges as the doctor's strongest – if not *only* – link to the event, and for this reason he must be provided with a very complete history. Often, of course, a child will realize that she has been stung only after the insect has flown away, so that visual identification of the offender is generally not possible. Nevertheless, information about the overall circumstances of the episode is immensely helpful. Such information may include any of the following facts:

> Where was the child when the sting occurred? Indoors? Outdoors? In the woods? In a flower garden? In a barn or on a picnic? Inside the house?

> Was there any evidence of a hive or nest nearby? If so, where was it located? Describe it in detail. Was there specific vegetation close by, such as rotting logs or an orchard in bloom?

> Were there any rubbish bags or open dustbins in the vicinity?

> Was the child stung more than once?

> Was a stinger found in the wound? Did you or the child attempt to remove it, and if so, how?

> What were the child's immediate symptoms? How long did it take for these symptoms to appear after the sting? Describe the progress and development of the symptoms in detail.

> How long did the symptoms last?

After a patient's history has been obtained, several laboratory tests may be in order. Standard testing procedures for insect stings include direct skin test methods and blood tests.

SKIN TESTS

Direct skin tests Direct skin tests are certainly the method of choice for the evaluation of aero-allergen (pollen) sensitivity; however, with *Hymenoptera* sensitivity this may not be the case. Direct skin tests for most insect allergy patients are an excellent method of establishing a diagnosis. For a small percentage of venom-sensitive children it may be necessary to perform a RAST test to confirm the diagnosis.

From a practical point of view it is necessary to wait at least two weeks after a suspected reaction has occurred before direct tests can be done. The testing will proceed in the usual manner of skin tests, beginning with an extremely diluted specific venom sample. The starting test dose will be 1/200,000th to 1/2,000,000th of the amount contained in a single sting. If the patient does not react to these low concentrations they will be gradually increased; the strongest dose is equal to 1/50th the strength of a usual sting. The testing procedure involves the use of both the prick/puncture and intracutaneous techniques (see pages 41–5 for details of these procedures).

Direct skin tests are highly accurate in confirming an allergic sensitivity to a specific insect. Their main drawback is that they are obviously performed directly on the patient. This can trigger a generalized reaction. In practice such reactions are extremely rare, and so far I have never encountered this problem.

BLOOD TESTS

Some physicians feel that the RAST test is a highly accurate method of testing for insect sting allergy. One drawback is the 15 to 20 per cent of false negative tests obtained by this technique. A false negative test is one that fails to show a positive reaction in someone who is truly allergic to a member of the *Hymenoptera*. A possible explanation for this response is felt to be an insufficient amount of IgE antibody circulating in the bloodstream. The direct skin test looks for IgE antibody which has already attached itself to the tissue mast cells.

One significant advantage of RAST over direct testing is that the patient doesn't run a risk of reacting to the RAST test. For the individual who had a severe anaphylactic reaction to the insect sting, the RAST test would probably be my first choice as a diagnostic procedure.

Another kind of blood test, not generally available and performed only in a few specialized research centres around the country, is the leucocyte histamine release procedure. Here a measurement is taken of the amount of histamine released by a patient's white blood cells when stimulated by a specific insect venom. This study is usually used to confirm a questionable direct or RAST test result.

RAST testing appears to be a good method of checking on the effectiveness of an immunotherapy programme. Your allergist may periodically perform this test to check how well your child is responding to this treatment.

WHOLE BODY EXTRACTS: A BRIEF NOTE OF WARNING

Until 1979 the only material available for the diagnosis and treatment of *Hymenoptera* sensitivity was known as whole body extract. This preparation was produced by pulverizing an insect, processing its remains, and producing a mixture composed of the entire body. The resulting whole body extract was then used to test and treat patients with *Hymenoptera* sensitivity. As you can imagine, much material in this final product was without therapeutic value of any kind. In a number of clinical studies it was proved that the use of whole body insect extract for both testing and treatment was ineffective and should be discontinued.

So if your child is currently being treated with whole body extracts, you should know that this procedure is decidedly out of date. In my opinion, your child should be retested for insect sensitivities using specific *Hymenoptera* venoms. If positive results are obtained, consideration should then be given to starting treatment with specific venom immunotherapy.

TREATMENT FOR INSECT STING ALLERGIES

There are three principal approaches to the treatment of insect sting allergies: preventive methods of avoiding insect stings, symptomatic medications for acute sting reactions, and immunotherapy.

PREVENTION OF STINGS

Of all allergic conditions, insect sting reactions may be the easiest to avoid. The process is simple: no contact; no sting; no reaction. Towards this aim the following suggestions are offered. No doubt you will have methods of your own to add to the list:

> The risk of being stung peaks in the late summer and early autumn, when *Hymenoptera* nests are particularly crowded and active.

> Make your child avoid areas where insects feed: orchards in bloom, clover fields, flower gardens, rubbish dumps, and picnic grounds.

> Do not let your child wear perfumes, colognes, scented deodorants and hair sprays.

> Make sure your child avoids playing or working in the garden near bushes, trees, stumps or any area where insect nests are usually found.

> If there is a nest on your property, have it removed by a professional. Call your local council if the offending nest is a beehive or a swarm of bees.

> Keep the windows of your car closed both when parked and when driving. Check the inside of the car for insects before getting in.

> Always make your child wear shoes when playing outdoors. Walking barefoot on a lawn or in a field is an invitation to a sting.

> Do not dress your child in loose-fitting clothes. These

may end up acting as a kind of net, entangling insects rather than protecting against them.

Always keep a can of insecticide in your home and car.

Do not dress your child in floral prints or highly coloured clothes; these patterns are especially attractive to flying insects.

If your child has already experienced a severe reaction to an insect sting, he should wear some type of identification tag describing the condition. A Medic Alert bracelet is excellent for this purpose. Parents are also well advised to keep an emergency insect sting kit on hand at all times. Prescriptions for these kits will be supplied by your doctor.

Learn and continually review the steps that must be taken in times of a sting emergency. Talk these steps over with your doctor until you are certain you understand everything involved: forewarned is forearmed.

MEDICAL TREATMENT FOR AN ACUTE STING

Treatment for an insect sting depends on the severity and nature of the sting itself. It is a question of degree.

A sting that does not cause an allergic reaction can be controlled by cleaning the area with alcohol and placing ice on the site to control swelling. If a stinger is protruding, flick it away with a knife blade or a fingernail. A standard home remedy for reducing pain is to mix baking soda with a small amount of water and apply it to the wound. All visible traces of the sting should be gone within a day or two.

For any generalized allergic reaction the most effective medication is adrenaline. If your child has had a generalized reaction to an insect sting, adrenaline is available in a pre-filled syringe called a Min-i-Jet. Your doctor should show you how to use it properly. You should also carry a small supply of antihistamine tablets and a dose should be taken at the same time.

Even if a sensitized child has been given an injection of

adrenaline at the sting site, she should still be rushed to hospital for observation. In most instances the only treatment will be an antihistamine given to control local swelling that persists even after the adrenaline has been administrered.

If the sting site becomes infected, it can easily be treated with appropriate antibiotics.

IMMUNOTHERAPY

While venom immunotherapy has been proved 96 to 98 per cent effective in preventing generalized allergic reactions to insect stings, it should be given only to individuals who meet *certain specific requirements*. (See page 61 for detailed information on immuno-therapy.) Exactly what these requirements are has been defined and redefined during the past decade as allergists have accumulated more and more case histories and as new research has been evalu-ated. Generally speaking, the two following conditions are necessary before venom immunotherapy should be recommended.

A documented history must exist of a generalized reaction to an insect sting. The reaction must have involved either the respir-atory and/or the cardiovascular system and have been serious enough to cause a drop in blood pressure (hypotension, fainting) or airway obstruction (swelling of the throat, difficulty in breathing, wheezing).

Positive test results must be obtained either by direct skin tests or the RAST technique. Negative test results combined with a positive medical history do *not* qualify a child as a candidate for immunotherapy.

When and if a positive history and confirming test results are obtained, the next step is to begin the venom immunotherapy injections. The usual schedule calls for weekly visits to the allergist for ten to fourteen weeks, then one visit every other week for two doses. Finally, a maintenance schedule consists of monthly visits. At the present time, maintenance programmes which extend the dosing period to once every six weeks or longer are being evalu-ated, and the reports so far seem very promising.

Currently, several researchers are studying RAST-deter-mined antibody levels as a possible method of predicting when it will be safe to discontinue immunotherapy. It is hoped that within a year or two we will be able to answer the constantly repeated question 'How much longer do I have to take these jabs?'

What side effects may occur from venom immunotherapy? Most patients experience no discomfort of any kind. When a reaction does occur it is almost always localized, consisting of redness, swelling and some immediate or delayed pain at the injection site. However, as previously mentioned, the subject of immunotherapy is in a state of change at the moment. It has virtually come to a halt because of the stringent precautions advised by the UK Committee on Safety of Medicines. This was brought about by a number of sudden deaths which were attributed to anaphylaxis, but there is hope that at some time in the future a measure of relaxation will come about which will allow this valuable prophylactic measure to be reintroduced.

NOTES ON OTHER INSECT PESTS

As an allergist I am also frequently asked if treatments exist to control 'allergic' reactions caused by flies and mosquitoes. First, let me say that these insects do not sting, they *bite*. In order to sting, a creature must have a stinger capable of injecting venom; neither flies nor mosquitoes possess such an apparatus. Moreover, the reaction following their bites is almost always local and almost never allergic. True, some children develop a very large swelling from mosquito bites, but this response is not an allergic one.

There have been reports of anaphylactic reactions following the bites of bedbugs and kissing bugs. These small, blood-sucking creatures work their mischief while their victims sleep and can indeed trigger a serious response, though only on the rarest occasions. The best method of controlling them is avoidance: increased personal hygiene and regular changing and laundering of the bedding are both mandatory.

The caterpillars of the brown-tail and yellow-tail moths are particularly allergenic. Although they are not very common, they can cause rashes if they are brought into contact with the skin. Avoidance is obviously the most effective measure.

Finally, general recommendations for the treatment of insect bites include the use of topical steroid creams to decrease itching and antihistamines such as Benadryl and Atarax for control of localized swelling. In the unlikely event that a generalized allergic reaction occurs, adrenaline is once again the best of all remedies. Unfortunately, at this time no forms of immunotherapy exist capable of controlling allergic reactions to insects outside the *Hymenoptera*.

QUESTIONS AND ANSWERS ON INSECT STING ALLERGIES

Is a child who has hay fever more likely to have an allergic reaction to an insect sting than a nonallergic child?

There is no evidence that I know of to indicate that a child with an allergic problem of *whatever* kind is more likely than a nonallergic child to develop insect sting sensitivities.

Is insect sting allergy inherited?

As far as we know, there is no indication of a hereditary pattern. If you or your parents, or your siblings, uncles and aunts for that matter, suffer from an insect sting allergy, you can rest assured that this in no way increases the chances of your own children developing such a problem.

Will the use of an insect repellent protect a child against the sting of a bee, wasp or hornet?

No. Repellent will sometimes keep flies, fleas and mosquitoes at bay. Against members of the *Hymenoptera* it is practically useless. Don't depend on it for that purpose.

How can you tell if a child is having an allergic reaction to an insect sting?

One simple method, as mentioned earlier, is to look for symptoms on the body distant from the sting site. For example, if a child is stung on the hand and develops an itchy rash on her chest, she is having an allergic reaction. If she is stung on the ear and develops difficulty catching her breath, it's the same thing.

> How soon after a person has been stung will an allergic reaction usually begin?

The answer depends on several factors. How allergic is the child? What part of the body was stung? Was the child stung more than once? While you will usually be able to identify a generalized anaphylactic reaction within the first few minutes after the sting, several hours may pass before any sign of reaction begins with ordinary allergic symptoms. Certainly it would be extremely unusual if any allergic symptoms took more than a twenty-four-hour period to appear.

> My daughter has been stung on two occasions by wasps. The second time her entire arm swelled up to twice its normal size. Should she be given immunotherapy for this reaction?

No, immunotherapy injections are not indicated for such local reactions, regardless of their severity. Recommendations for treatment are made only if a child shows a generalized reaction with evidence of breathing difficulty, a drop in blood pressure or a loss of consciousness.

CHAPTER NINE

Food Allergies

An area of particular frustration for parents and allergists alike is the murky, unpredictable world of food allergies. If you listen to the many 'experts' holding forth on radio and TV today or if you read certain pseudoscientific publications lining the pop book-shelves, you may already believe that food allergies are as common as headaches or that they produce a range of symptoms that run the gamut from anxiety to arthritis. We are told by these 'experts' that children who are bothered by insomnia, who have discipline problems or trouble concentrating in class, are actually suffering from an allergy to some unnamed antigen in their morning cereal or to a chemical in their school lunch. Some doctors go so far as to say that they possess infallible diagnostic methods by which they can magically determine which foods are causing the troublesome symptoms and then clear the whole thing up tidily with appro-priate diet therapy.

I only wish these claims were true and that it was possible to resolve such problems by merely regulating your child's menu. But the food allergy question is far more complicated and unde-fined than certain elements of the lay press would have you believe, and allergists are still groping for fundamental answers. In this chapter you will learn the crucial things we *do* know about food allergies and, perhaps more importantly, you will find out what workable therapies exist to control them.

FOOD ALLERGY VERSUS FOOD INTOLERANCE

While the actual incidence of food allergy among children is very difficult to determine, there are unquestionably fewer cases than some doctors and lay preachers would have us believe. Many reactions labelled allergic later turn out to stem from other causes. At this point, before things get too confused, let's define and explain our terms.

Food allergy reaction Allergic reactions to food develop *only* when an individual becomes sensitized to a particular food. This means that specific antibodies (IgE class proteins) have been produced, indicating that the child is now sensitized. Each time the youngster is given that food – egg, for example – an allergic reaction will take place, causing chemical mediators to be released into the bloodstream. These chemical mediators – histamine being the most familiar – then produce the spectrum of allergic symptoms. These symptoms may involve not only the intestinal tract where the food is digested (vomiting, diarrhoea) but also the skin (hives, eczema) and the lungs (asthma). A person highly allergic to a food can have an anaphylactic reaction after eating a small amount of that food (see page 13 for a complete description of the allergic triggering process).

Food intolerance reaction Clinically, a food intolerance is often mistaken for an allergic response. However, from a theoretical point of view the two are fundamentally different. A food intolerance reaction does not involve allergic sensitization; there is therefore no production of IgE antibodies within the bloodstream. Let's look at some of the prominent factors that trigger this response.

Food poisoning This type of response occurs as a result of the direct action of either the food or an additive chemical. It does not involve an allergic or immune reaction. Symptoms occur because of toxins (poisons) released by bacteria or parasites that have contaminated the food.

Anaphylactoid reaction Whenever there is a generalized release of chemical mediators in the body that is not caused by an allergic triggering response, we have what is known as an anaphylactoid reaction. This reaction produces generalized intestinal, respiratory and skin responses which by all outward signs appear to be the same as those typical of an anaphylactic reaction; yet, to stress the fact again, this response is *not* induced by allergic causes. Anaphylactoid reactions can occur after the ingestion of foods which contain large amounts of the chemical histamine, such as tuna fish, mackerel and Swiss cheese.

Metabolic food reaction This response is triggered by food substances that have an adverse affect on a child's normal metabolism. Symptoms include diarrhoea, cramps and bloating, all of which can occur within the first few weeks of an infant's life. As a rule, such reactions are experienced by individuals who are already weakened by malnutrition, disease or medicines that affect normal metabolic functions.

A good example of a metabolic food reaction is the inherited absence of an enzyme in the system called lactase, a substance necessary for the proper digestion of lactose. Children born with this condition cannot digest dairy products – lactose is the milk sugar found in most dairy products – and hence must be fed milk substitutes such as soy formula. Some population groups appear to be at greater risk than others. Among North American blacks, for instance, 70 to 80 per cent suffer from bowel wall lactase deficiency, while 55 to 95 per cent of Asians have the same problem. Contrast these figures with the low 5 to 20 per cent incidence in North American Caucasians, or with the 3 per cent incidence among Danish children. If a child has lactose intolerance the condition will usually reveal itself early in life, sometimes during the first weeks. Parents of newborn babies should be on the alert for this problem, and should quickly seek a doctor's advice if their child seems unable to tolerate a milk-based formula.

RECOGNIZING THE SYMPTOMS OF FOOD ALLERGY

If it is indeed so difficult to recognize and diagnose food allergies, what symptoms, if any, can be considered at least suggestive of an allergic food reaction?

From one standpoint the answer is that no single symptom or even pattern of symptoms offers foolproof evidence. In fact, the only way to diagnose a food allergy properly is by careful observation of *all* symptoms, even those which do not originate in the gastrointestinal tract. However, at the same time, the two systems where allergic symptoms caused by food sensitivity are most likely to occur are the gastrointestinal tract and the skin.

GASTROINTESTINAL SYMPTOMS

Any child who ingests a food to which he is allergic may develop immediate symptoms that can start with an itching sensation of the lips. This reaction is frequently followed by localized swelling of the lips, mouth and tongue; occasionally the swelling becomes so severe that it obstructs the breathing tubes and impairs breathing, creating a life-threatening situation. One young patient of mine had a reaction of this kind every time she ate cashew nuts. Another developed difficulty breathing whenever he ate eggs or lobster.

As we progress deeper into the gastrointestinal tract, the primary symptoms are cramping abdominal pain accompanied by nausea, vomiting and diarrhoea. A list of the most common gastrointestinal reactions includes:

swelling of the tongue and throat

localized itching of the lips and mouth

difficulty in swallowing

nausea and vomiting

general abdominal pain and 'stomach ache'

diarrhoea

itching of the anal area

bleeding from the small and large intestine (unusual)

SYMPTOMS OF THE SKIN

Though often difficult to pinpoint, food allergies are one of the principal causes of hives and angioedema among younger children. Eggs, dairy products and wheat are the main offenders here, though foods such as nuts (including peanuts), shellfish, chocolate and berries may contribute as well. No part of the body is immune from food-induced hives or angioedema. Typical allergic responses of the skin include:

itching

redness and burning of the skin

hives and/or angioedema

atopic dermatitis

OTHER AREAS WHERE FOOD-ALLERGIC SYMPTOMS MAY APPEAR

Some children develop coughing and wheezing as the result of food allergies. The incidence of asthma attacks triggered by a specific food sensitivity, however, is not very high, and when it does occur it is usually obvious which food is to blame. The most common offenders in this instance are milk and other dairy products, followed by corn, peanuts and eggs.

An allergic food reaction may also trigger such classically allergic symptoms as sneezing, runny nose, weeping, red and swollen eyes, shortness of breath, rapid heartbeat, shock and collapse. These signs occur singly or, on rare occasions, all at once, in which case a severe generalized allergic response is at work: anaphylaxis. A food reaction of this intensity is rare, but when it occurs it is a *medical emergency* and requires medical attention.

Finally, some doctors feel that a variety of symptoms such as hyperactivity, joint pains, bedwetting, insomnia, fatigue, migraine headaches, anxiety, muscular aches, depression, and arthritis are caused by food allergies. This notion is based on what I consider to be inadequate evidence, as many of the procedures used to document the 'allergic' nature of these symptoms – and many of the methods employed to treat them – can at best be described as controversial. (A discussion of unproven diagnostic and therapeutic techniques in treating allergies will be found in the chapter 'Parents Beware'.)

FOODS MOST LIKELY TO TRIGGER ALLERGIC REACTIONS

This rather lengthy list begins with the first food for most of us: milk.

Cow's milk Most infants who are not breastfed are initially fed with a formula derived from cow's milk. Since an infant's intestinal tract is still relatively immature, milk proteins can easily pass through the intestinal wall and react with cells of the immune system, thus getting an early start on allergic sensitization. Milk allergy, as a result, is one of the most frequent and early of all food problems. Its symptoms run the gamut from nasal congestion, to severe vomiting and chronic diarrhoea, to allergic skin rashes such as atopic dermatitis and hives. It can be caused by dairy products of all kinds including cheese, ice cream, ice milk, yogurt and butter as well as foods containing milk solids, casein, caseinate and lactalbumin.

What should you do about milk allergies? Eliminate milk and milk products from your child's diet. The organizations listed on page 320 will be able to help with information. Better yet, most children who develop dairy allergies outgrow them after several years. In my experience the great majority of children who are allergic to cow's milk during the first one to two years of life come to tolerate it quite nicely by the time they are five to seven years old.

Cereal grains This very common food group is found in an almost limitless number of preparations we eat on a daily basis. The major representatives are wheat, corn, millet, rye, oats, barley and rice. Of the seven, wheat and corn are by far the most frequent and serious offenders. Allergic symptoms triggered by grain tend to involve the gastrointestinal tract, producing nausea, vomiting, abdominal pains and diarrhoea, though symptoms such as rhinitis, asthma and hives can also occur.

One of the hazards of cereal allergies is that both wheat and corn are 'hidden' in many common foods, especially corn in the form of cornstarch or corn sweeteners. Watch out for the following commercial food items, all of which contain one or both of these grains:

baked beans (corn)
candy bars (corn/wheat)
beer (corn)
chewing gum (corn)
corn oil
glue on envelopes and
  stamps (corn)
ketchup (corn)
marshmallows (corn)
mayonnaise (corn)

popcorn
salad dressing (corn
gravy (wheat/corn)
ice cream cones (corn/wheat)
luncheon meats (wheat/corn)
coffee substitute (wheat)
fried chicken (wheat)
hot dogs (wheat)
macaroni, spaghetti and all
  forms of pasta (wheat)

These hidden sources can in most instances be avoided by scrutinizing food labels and avoiding any products that contain the offending substances. If you have any questions, contact the manufacturers directly.

What about rye? Is it a good substitute for wheat bread? Because an all-rye bread won't rise, from 40 to 60 per cent of all rye bread recipes call for wheat flour in addition to the rye. A 100 per cent rye bread is available but hard to find. The best bet is the bakery shelves of a natural foods store, or better yet, your own home oven.

Citrus fruits The citrus family includes oranges, tangerines, grapefruits, lemons, limes, kumquats and a few other fruits. Many children develop allergic intestinal symptoms from these foods, especially from orange juice. Contact dermatitis is a local inflammatory, irritative skin reaction that can occur after many substances, including foods, cosmetics and certain types of jewellery, touch the skin. This type of response may develop around the mouth when a citrus food comes in contact with the area. Some youngsters can tolerate small amounts of citrus juices, especially if the juice is watered down and not consumed on a daily basis. Be aware that some forms of fruit punch or fruit drink such as grape or apple may contain citrus juices hidden in the mixture and are a potential source of trouble.

Chocolate Of all the foods we have mentioned, chocolate is undoubtedly the least essential for children *and* the most difficult to prevent them from eating. A related member of this food family is the cola nut; hence cola drinks such as Coke, Pepsi and Dr Pepper should be eliminated from the diet of any child with a chocolate sensitivity.

The following substances infrequently cause allergic reactions:

apples or apple juice	pears
bananas	plums
barley	potatoes
beef	rice
beets	rye
carrots	salt
grape juice	soybean milk
lamb	spring water
lettuce	sweet potatoes
marrow	tea
oats	turkey
peaches	

These substances *most often* cause allergic reactions:

chocolate	nuts
eggs	pork
fish	shellfish
fresh fruit, especially berries	tomato products
milk	

EVALUATING FOOD ALLERGIES

Your visit to an allergist will be especially productive if you come prepared to answer specific questions concerning your child's condition. Typical of a doctor's queries are the following:

What specific food-related symptoms have you observed? Describe in as much detail as you can the pattern of these symptoms.

When do symptoms occur in relation to meals?

How long do these symptoms last?

Have the allergic patterns changed since you first began to notice them? In what ways?

Does the child have any particular food cravings? Does she actively avoid certain foods? Which ones?

What treatment, if any, has been used to relieve the symptoms? How successful has it been?

Are you suspicious of a specific food or food group such as dairy products, egg-containing substances or citrus fruits? On what evidence is your suspicion based?

What foods does your child normally eat? Give sample breakfast, lunch and dinner menus. Information on the child's favourite foods, her snacking patterns, the amounts of food the child eats, will all be helpful.

For an infant, all facts regarding formula will be crucial. So will all recent changes in the diet and information on the child's general eating patterns, the sequence of new foods recently introduced to the diet and the kinds of vitamins being taken.

Are other members of the child's family allergic to any particular foods? Which ones? Is there allergy of any kind in your family? If so, describe it.

What is your child's general allergic history, if any? Is the child currently being treated for other allergic problems?

Describe your child's physical growth history. If possible, provide height and weight charts. These will be evaluated to determine if she is developing normally.

If your child vomits frequently, how soon after eating does the vomiting take place? Describe the appearance of the vomited material.

How often does the child have a bowel movement? Is the stool usually well formed or is it watery, hard, loose, bloody? Does it have any unusual odour?

This list is, of course, only a sampling of the many possible questions that will be reviewed in depth. The child's medical and allergic history is the allergist's single most effective diagnostic tool.

Following the taking of the history, a complete physical examination will be performed. The doctor will be looking for typical signs and symptoms of allergy such as skin rashes, dark circles under the eyes, nasal congestion and wheezing. In addition, the doctor will make a general assessment of your child's nutritional condition: how good is the muscle tone? Is the child overweight or underweight?

Following the examination the allergist must then decide which tests, if any, are required to complete the evaluation. General screening procedures that may be called for include:

A serum IgE level test IgE is the specific protein elevated in the bloodstream of patients who are either actively allergic or who have a tendency in this direction. When a high IgE level is present, it is a strong indication that the patient is allergy-prone. (See page 37 for further discussion of the IgE level.)

Skin tests Direct skin tests using the prick/puncture technique (see pages 42–3) are the best screening method we have today for evaluating a patient suspected of having a food allergy. Despite this statement, I have not been impressed with any type of direct testing procedure when it comes to the question of food allergy. There are many problems associated with skin testing for food. Let me illustrate just one type of problem the allergist has to cope with: false-positive and false-negative food test results. Here are two examples: Tony, aged four, was suspected of developing hives whenever he ate food containing tomatoes. Since pizza was his favourite food, it became very important to find out if he really was allergic. The prick test for tomato was negative. On his next visit, Tony was only too happy to devour a tomato, and within thirty minutes the hives appeared. This is an illustration of a false-negative test result.

On the other hand, Cindy, a nine-year-old, had been denied the pleasure of eating chocolate for many weeks. Her mother suspected that Cindy's stomach pains developed whenever she drank Coca-Cola or ate a chocolate bar. Her test was positive. When she was challenged with increasing amounts of cola drinks and chocolate over several days there was absolutely no discomfort. So here we have a false-positive test result.

Unfortunately, these situations occur all too frequently in the evaluation of patients suspected of having a food allergy. While these procedures may be of assistance for a small number of patients, the personal history remains the single most effective method of diagnosis.

RAST test This is an in vitro laboratory test that has been used quite often in the evaluation of patients suspected of having food allergy. I believe that often this test is ordered very unselectively. While an occasional patient will be an appropriate candidate for it, most of the time I have found that the results contradicted the history. This serves to confuse rather than clarify the picture.

MANAGEMENT OF FOOD ALLERGIES

In my opinion, and in the opinion of many allergists today, the best method for both diagnosing and treating reactions to food is by dietary manipulation. What does this term mean? More or less what it implies is the addition and removal of both natural and artificial substances from the diet, both for the purpose of diagnosing and treating symptoms caused by a suspected food or foods. Here are some of the dietary manipulation techniques I have found most effective.

Keeping a food diary Any parent whose child is suspected of having a food allergy should make use of a basic food diary. This is done by keeping a detailed list of *all* the foods and beverages – even medications and substances such as toothpaste and mouthwash – taken by the patient in the course of a day. Preferably in a notebook that is kept handy day and night, the diary serves as an ongoing record of everything that has passed the child's lips at a friend's house, for lunch, dinner, snacks, at school, in front of the TV, on a hike, before bed, at the cinema, whatever.

For how many days or weeks should the diary be kept? It depends on the frequency of the complaints. If your child has suspected food-related symptoms every day, then a diary which covers a seven-to-ten-day period will be adequate. If the problem occurs once every five to seven days, then at least a month must be spent in compiling the record.

At the end of the designated time, you and your doctor will examine the diary to see if any identifiable patterns are present. If it is impossible to draw conclusions, there is no reason to continue with the diary. If, on the other hand, there is a suggestion that a specific food might be causing the symptoms, an elimination diet is the next step. An explanation of that procedure follows.

This diary approach is, of course, entirely dependent on the thoroughness of the parents' record-keeping, the frequency with which the child's symptoms occur, and the doctor's ability to discern a pattern in the compiled data. Table 10 shows how a sample page of a food diary might appear.

Diet restriction Certain foods are more likely than others to provoke allergic reactions in children. Highest on the list are milk, chocolate (including cola drinks), corn, citrus fruits, eggs, wheat, nuts, fish with scales, and shellfish. If you suspect that these or some other foods in particular are causing the problem, and if the symptoms occur frequently, or better yet if they are present every day, you can try for a limited time to be your own doctor. While this evaluation must be done at home, it is best practised under medical guidance.

Start by removing the food in question and any substances which contain this food from your child's diet for a period of seven to fourteen days. During this time see if the suspicious symptom has disappeared. Within a week or two you should be able to tell whether the suspected food is at fault, simply because its absence from the menu should coincide with the absence of the symptoms.

Table 10   Sample Diary Entry

Date	Time food was eaten	Type of food	Reactions, if any
15/2			
	7.00 A.M.	Brushed teeth with Colgate	None
	7.15	Cornflakes with milk and apple slices	None
		Orange juice	None
	10.30	Milk and biscuits	Slight stomach ache
	12.30 P.M.	Spaghetti and meat sauce	None
		White bread and butter	None
		Glass of milk	None
	4.45	Chocolate bar	None
	6.30	Roast beef	None
		Gravy	None
		Peas	None
		Chips	None
		Glass of chocolate milk	None
	7.45	Biscuits and Ovaltine	None
	8.00	Brushed teeth with Colgate	None

Next, reintroduce the food, beginning with very small portions (that is to say, half an ounce of milk, a sixth of an egg yolk) and increase the amount every day until you are giving a regular portion. If the symptoms return, the diagnostic battle is three-quarters won. To win it entirely, repeat the same process once more, making sure not to change any of the variables. If the results can be duplicated *twice*, you may be certain you have discovered the culprit. If, on the other hand, the removal of the tested food has no effect on the symptoms one way or the other, acquit this substance and go on to another. This technique is called an *elimination diet*. If symptoms occur infrequently, it may not be feasible to use this technique for diagnosis.

General comments Foods that cause hives and those that may cause 'allergic reactions' are not necessarily synonymous. A child may develop symptoms of sneezing, runny nose, cough, wheeze, nausea or vomiting as a consequence of an allergic reaction to food. They may never exhibit any skin symptoms such as atopic dermatitis (an eczematous eruption), itching or the appearance of hives.

There is nothing wrong with a short-term do-it-yourself diet manipulation. The removal of a food or food group (i.e. dairy or citrus) from the diet for seven to fourteen days will not cause any significant nutritional disturbance. The only time there is any danger is when the initial reaction suspected of being triggered by a food was anaphylactic. I don't believe that in this situation any parent should ever be his or her own doctor!

Food challenge test The only way to be completely certain that a particular food is causing a specific symptom is to eat that food and observe the results. The most controlled method we have for doing this is the double-blind food challenge test. Here neither the doctor nor the patient knows whether the substance about to be eaten is the suspected food or a placebo. If, for example, it is suspected that Elizabeth is getting hives from peanuts and if her symptoms have continued for several years, it is conceivable that if she just *thinks* she is going to eat peanuts an attack will occur. If no one, neither patient nor doctor, knows whether the substance about to be eaten contains peanuts or a tolerated food, the results will be uninfluenced either by suggestion or expectation.

As a rule, challenge tests are done in hospitals or in a doctor's surgery where emergency measures are available in case reactions turn out to be unexpectedly severe. The test food is freeze-dried to disguise its taste. It is fed to the child in an opaque capsule and the child is observed for the presence or absence of symptoms. Children too young to swallow capsules are given small amounts of the suspected substance hidden in tolerated foods.

Once challenge or elimination techniques have determined that a food allergy actually exists, treatment consists of avoiding the offending substance and its entire family of related foods. For example, if a child is allergic to milk she must also avoid butter, cream, yogurt, cheese, ice cream and milk solids in other foods. Does this mean that Susie can never eat peanut butter again, or eggs? In general, no. For most children food allergies are temporary, and except in the rare situation in which an anaphylactic reaction occurred, the cautious reintroduction of an eliminated food may begin within six to twelve months after its removal. Before taking such a step, of course, a discussion with your doctor is in order. In general, the earlier in life the problem is detected, the greater the chances are that the specific sensitivity will disappear.

OTHER POSSIBLE TREATMENTS FOR FOOD ALLERGIES

Other forms of treatment for food problems are considerably less effective than diet regulation. Sodium cromoglycate, a drug commonly prescribed for asthma and rhinitis (see the chapters on asthma and rhinitis), has been given by mouth in an attempt to treat food allergies. The amounts that must be used, however, are large and the results have not been impressive. For this purpose, sodium cromoglycate comes in the form of capsules under the brand name of Nalcrom.

Research, of course, continues on other drugs which may some day prove helpful, but to date none is ready for clinical trials. Immunotherapy and oral desensitization have from time to time been prescribed for this problem but from my experience, and the experience of most other allergists, they are not recommended for routine clinical use.

FOOD ADDITIVES AND ALLERGY

Chemical substances that colour, preserve, and stabilize are being added to our foods in ever-increasing numbers. While these agents are supposed to improve the condition and prolong the freshness of our food supply, they have also been responsible for causing a large number of harmful side effects. Some of these reactions can be classified as idiosyncratic or unusual; others are truly allergic.

One of the major offenders in this group is a dye called tartrazine, known by the code number E102. However, all the colourings which come under the headings of azo dyes and coal tar dyes are also suspect and adverse reactions in sensitized children have been attributed to them. See Appendix.

Monosodium glutamate (MSG, code no. 621), which is used

both as a flavouring agent and a meat tenderizer, is responsible for the condition known as the Chinese Restaurant Syndrome. Typical symptoms include headache, facial flushing, and chest pain.

Sodium benzoate, a preservative, has been reported to cause severe asthma symptoms in adults. It has rarely been responsible for causing problems for children.

Sensitivity to sulphites is becoming a significant problem for both paediatric and adult asthma patients. Since the late 1970s more and more fresh, frozen, and processed foods have been preserved with a variety of sulphiting agents. These include sodium bisulphite, sodium metabisulphite, and sulphur dioxide.

With the trend towards eating natural or healthy foods, more of us are heading for the salad bars found in many restaurants. Unfortunately the sulphiting chemicals are used to preserve the freshness of many of the vegetables at the salad bar.

The most significant reactions caused by sulphite sensitivity are severe asthma and anaphylactic shock.

Clearly, while additives are not a major cause of allergic difficulties in children, their potential to cause adverse reactions has been well documented. Since 1 January 1986, additives (with the exceptions of flavourings) are either listed with the ingredients on the label by name or under 'E' numbers. The 'E' numbers were introduced so that foods could be moved from country to country within the European Common Market. Numbers without the 'E' are sometimes encountered.

Leaflets giving the list of 'E' numbers and what they mean can be obtained from the Ministry of Agriculture or from the Food and Drink Federation. (See Appendix for addresses.)

THE FEINGOLD HYPOTHESIS

A discussion of the ill effects of chemical allergens would not be complete without a word regarding the famous Feingold hypothesis. In 1975, Dr Benjamin Feingold wrote a book proclaiming that artificial dyes, colourings and food preservatives can often be the unsuspected cause of hyperactivity in children. If a child is placed on a diet free of these potentially harmful chemical substances, Feingold maintained, these hyperactive behaviour patterns will soon disappear.

Extensive publicity in the lay press and on TV quickly followed Dr Feingold's book, and for a while the Feingold diet was extremely popular, even though the programme it called for required a considerable investment of time, effort and expense. The only problem with this highly attractive hypothesis was that it simply did not hold up when rigidly controlled scientific evaluations of Dr Feingold's theories were carried out in independent medical centres throughout the country.

What is the current thinking about Dr Feingold's hypothesis? Most allergists would agree that only a very small percentage of hyperactive children might benefit from a rigidly maintained diet free of all artificial colouring, dyes and other additives. However, the time, effort and expense involved in attempting to continue such a programme over a long period (possibly years) does not make this approach a reasonable option for most families. The success rate for this diet is somewhere between 5 and 10 per cent. Based on what I have said, I do not recommend this approach for my patients.

Summing Up

Despite advances in the diagnosis of suspected food allergies using such procedures as RAST testing and double-blind food challenges, clinical allergy still has some way to go before this complicated and frustrating problem can be entirely solved. However, new diagnostic techniques are constantly being evaluated that should provide us with the necessary tools to diagnose the problem accurately and treat it successfully. Meanwhile, with an approach on the part of the parents that is based on common sense and carried out in a logical step-by-step fashion, the great majority of children can now be helped, some to the extent that they can be kept largely symptom free.

QUESTIONS AND ANSWERS ABOUT FOOD ALLERGIES

At what age may parents begin to see symptoms of food allergies in their child?

Once a child has been exposed to a food and has become sensitized to it, allergic symptoms can begin at any time. This means that foods eaten by the mother during pregnancy could conceivably sensitize the child. I have seen children display allergic reactions to their formula within the first few days of life.

Is it possible to eat a certain food for a long period of time and then suddenly become allergic to it?

Yes, a child can become allergic to a food today that she tolerated yesterday. It's a question really of how long it takes to become sensitized. For some children this process occurs after a short exposure; for others it may require years.

A child who has a severe allergic reaction to a specific food inadvertently eats this food. What should be done?

Make him vomit immediately so that all the offending food is removed from his intestinal tract. Then give him an antihistamine. Watch the child carefully for the development of symptoms. If intestinal, skin or respiratory discomfort is noted, take him to the nearest doctor or hospital for observation and possible treatment.

What relationship, if any, exists between migraine headaches and food allergies?

There does seem to be a small but definite segment of young migraine patients who suffer from food sensitivity.

Does cooked food tend to cause fewer allergic problems than raw food?

As a general rule, cooked food is less likely to trigger an

allergic response than the same food uncooked. This is especially true of fruits and vegetables.

Can touching or smelling a food trigger an allergic reaction in a sensitized child?

Yes, it is possible for a young person who is highly allergic to develop symptoms merely by contact or inhalation. I once treated a three-year-old girl who was so egg-sensitive she would break out with generalized hives whenever she touched an egg, even if the egg was still in its shell. I also know of a four-year-old boy who developed severe asthmatic symptoms the moment he entered a house or restaurant where the odour of cooked fish was in the air. Such sensitivities are rare.

Are food allergies seasonal?

The only way in which the time of year might play a role is if a child has a seasonal allergy problem such as rose or hay fever. Then, when the child experiences symptoms of the seasonal allergy, the eating of a food normally tolerated during a period of acute allergic symptoms may prove just the straw to break the camel's back, causing the child to react allergically to the food as well. It might also be pointed out that fruits and vegetables are by their nature seasonal. While it appears to Johnny's parents that Johnny suffers from allergies only in the late summer, this problem is actually caused (for the sake of argument) by the fact that fresh peaches, the real source of the problem, are available only at that time of year.

Can a person be allergic to common seasonings such as salt and pepper?

Pepper, along with the array of spices commonly used in our daily diet, can occasionally cause allergic problems. So can the chemical flavouring MSG (monosodium glutamate), which many cooks use to tenderize meat and enhance the flavour of vegetables. As far as I know – though anything is possible in this field – salt by itself has never been responsible for any such difficulties.

Are all foods capable of causing allergies?

While there are some foods which are quite unlikely to provoke allergic reactions such as veal and rice, there is no single substance which is totally safe. The fact is that at some time someone somewhere will develop a reaction to even the most 'nonallergic' food.

Do labels on a food product list all the ingredients found in that item?

Yes, except for flavourings. Since 1 January 1986 all foods contain in the list of ingredients the additives, either by name or under the 'E' number. A leaflet can be obtained to decode the 'E' numbers. (See Appendix for addresses.)

My six-month-old cannot tolerate either cow's milk or soy formula. What other choices are there?

There is a variety of specialized formulas on the market. Nutramigen (Mead Johnson) and Vivonex (Norwich Eaton) contain primary essential amino acids. These require special preparation instructions and must be recommended by your doctor.

Does a nursing mother need to watch the foods she is eating?

Definitely. Any food a mother eats will soon appear in her breast milk, even if only in small amounts. Children who are sensitized to a specific food can develop allergic symptoms this way. Nursing mothers should *always* be aware and careful of the foods they eat.

CHAPTER TEN
Adverse Drug Reactions

While accurate figures are difficult to obtain, it has been estimated that as many as 30 per cent of hospitalized patients experience some type of adverse reaction to the drugs they receive. Even if these figures are a little high, the possibility of developing a drug reaction must be considered whenever a prescription is written.

What, it might then be asked, does the expression 'adverse drug reaction' actually mean? Specifically, it *is a response to a drug that involves unexpected, unwanted, unpleasant symptoms.* Though many people tend to think of adverse drug reactions as being allergic, the truth is that they can stem from a variety of causes of which allergic response is just one. A comprehensive list of causes includes:

allergic reaction

intolerance

idiosyncratic reactions

overdose

side effects

drug interactions

psychogenic responses

The following imaginary conversation between a doctor and a parent is a very common occurrence.

MRS JOHNSON: Doctor Smith, Sally has been taking penicillin now for five days – like you told her – and she's developed a bad rash.

DR SMITH: Where's the rash located? What colour is it?

MRS JOHNSON: It's red, and it's all over her arms and legs.

DR SMITH: Sounds like an allergy. Stop the medication right away. Sally should keep away from penicillin entirely from now on. It could be serious! I'll prescribe a different antibiotic.

In the future, penicillin may again be indicated for Sally. But when another doctor attempts to prescribe it Sally's mother will no doubt protest, regaling the doctor with horror stories of how poor Sally broke out so badly with that 'allergic rash' last time she took penicillin, and how her former doctor warned that penicillin could be dangerous.

In my experience, Sally's rash and a large number of other suspected drug reactions can and often do stem from nonallergic causes. The entire subject of allergic reactions to drugs is extremely frustrating because medical technology has not yet developed accurate tests to prove whether a person is or isn't truly allergic to a specific drug. There is, however, one significant exception to this statement, and that is our ability to diagnose penicillin allergy. The point to be made here is that a diagnosis of drug allergy should not be made automatically simply from a description given over the phone. Only after a complete study should a doctor diagnose a specific drug allergy.

Since we are currently not able to test accurately for possible allergy to most drugs, this diagnosis should be made after consideration has been given to *all* clinical possibilities. For example, 5 to 15 per cent of patients who take a form of penicillin called Ampicillin will develop a generalized rash that is *not* an allergic reaction. If possible, the doctor should examine all patients suspected of having drug reactions while physical evidence of the suspected reaction is still present. Using this information, along with the history and results of the physical examination, he may be able to diagnose the cause of the reaction *without* misleading the parents concerning a nonexistent allergy.

THE MANY CAUSES OF DRUG REACTIONS

Since the difference between allergic and nonallergic drug reactions is so important for parents to understand, let's examine in detail the different types of reactions.

Allergic drug reactions Before a drug allergy manifests itself – a reaction to penicillin, let us say – a child must first produce specific anti-IgE antibodies against that drug – i.e. *anti-penicillin IgE antibodies*. These special proteins will be found on the tissue mast cells and the basophils circulating in the bloodstream of a child who has broken out with generalized hives after taking penicillin. These antibodies can be produced only when a child has been exposed and sensitized to the specific drug. (For a complete discussion of IgE and the sensitization process, see page 20.)

Having read this statement, you may protest that your child had an allergic reaction the very first time she ever took a particular medicine. It might seem that this was the cause, but your child could have been exposed to the particular drug in question without anyone ever realizing it. For example, when a nursing mother is taking a particular medication, minute amounts of the drug are passed from her breast milk to the child. Antibiotics are occasionally put into animal feed to prevent disease. Small amounts of these substances can then pass into our food chain and hence into the child's diet. These are only two – among many – possible sources of hidden exposure.

True allergic reactions to drugs occur in only a small percentage of the general population. There appears to be no relationship between a child's allergic reactions to things such as dust and pollen and the tendency to develop drug allergies. Even if six-year-old Andrew suffers from serious hay fever or eczema, he is, statistically speaking, no more likely to develop drug reactions than ten-year-old Louise, who has never been allergic to anything in her life.

Six-year-old Ruth was given penicillin three times in her infancy and experienced no problems. The fourth time she developed serious allergic symptoms and had to be rushed to hospital. In other words, a child who is potentially sensitive to a particular drug may have taken it on several previous occasions without experiencing any allergic response. The time it takes to become sensitized to a specific medication varies greatly from child to child.

Once your child is sensitized, allergic drug reactions generally occur within twenty-four hours after the drug has been taken, though delayed reactions are not unusual. As a rule, the more severe an allergic drug reaction, the more rapid the onset of symptoms will be. An anaphylactic reaction, the most severe form of generalized allergic response, almost always begins within the first thirty to sixty minutes after the medicine enters the body. Allergic skin rashes, on the other hand, may sometimes develop as late as six or seven days after the child has taken the drug.

Once a child is sensitized to a particular drug, even minute amounts of it can trigger a reaction.

A child who develops allergic symptoms to one drug is likely to react in a similar way to other drugs derived from the same chemical family. This is particularly true of penicillin-related preparations.

Symptoms of allergic drug reactions usually subside within four to six days after the drug has been discontinued. On infrequent occasions a drug reaction may continue for many weeks. In extremely rare cases it may last for months.

Tests for penicillin and insulin sensitivity are after-the-fact procedures – there are no reliable *prospective* testing methods currently available – and screening procedures for drug allergy in general are at present quite limited. The ultimate test is to readminister the drug to the child and note its effects. This type of challenge test is of course potentially *quite dangerous*; if it is to be considered at all, it must be done in a medical setting where treatment for a severe reaction can be given quickly. In most instances it is unnecessary to perform this risky procedure. Later in this chapter I will discuss specific desensitization techniques that offer another alternative.

The route by which a drug enters the body – by mouth, injection or topically through the skin – is a critical factor in determining whether that drug will cause allergic sensitization. Topical application is the route most likely to produce sensitization. Oral administration, perhaps surprisingly, is the least likely. Topical preparations containing antibiotics and antihistamines are especially prone to cause problems, and at present a number of over-the-counter preparations include *both* classes of drugs. Do not use them indiscriminately. Talk to your doctor if you have any questions.

Intolerance First on the list of nonallergic drug reactions is a condition known as drug intolerance. Simply stated, drug intolerance refers to an unexpected increase in the *usual* activity of a drug. For example, we know that if double or triple the average dose of aspirin is taken for several days, almost everyone will develop tinnitus, more commonly known as a ringing in the ears. Someone who is intolerant of aspirin would develop tinnitus after taking only one or two aspirin tablets, a normal dose. What we have is a quantitative increase in the pharmacological action of the drug. There is no way to predict whether or not this type of reaction will occur.

Generally speaking, there is no way to control drug intolerance. Some children just can't tolerate any amount of a certain drug. A substitute preparation will have to be prescribed.

Idiosyncratic drug response If Jenny takes an aspirin to relieve her headache and develops a blood condition called haemolytic anaemia, she has had an idiosyncratic reaction: an unexpected effect that is different from the normal action of the drug. Such responses occur only in a susceptible population – the likelihood of many people developing them is small – and most symptoms are based on an unusual metabolic response rather than an immune one. Medications that produce idiosyncratic responses should *never* be given to susceptible patients, even in the smallest doses.

Drug overdose Allergic drug reactions, drug intolerance and drug idiosyncrasy occur only among people who have a biological tendency to develop such conditions. The symptoms of drug overdose require no such predisposing susceptibility: it can happen to anyone, on purpose or by accident. The symptoms are toxic, not allergic, and can range from uncomfortable to fatal. The problem is avoided by monitoring drug intake, by careful medicating procedures, and by keeping all medicine away from very young children. Always read medication instructions carefully and ask your doctor about the medicines prescribed for your child.

Side effects of drugs We are all familiar with the phenomenon of side effects, those unwanted extra symptoms which accompany the expected pharmacological activity of a drug. A frequent example is the headache, jittery feeling, tremor and rapid heartbeat that follow an injection of adrenaline for acute asthma. Side effects are the most common form of adverse drug reactions, more frequent by far than either drug intolerance or allergy. Many people come into my consulting room and tell me they are allergic to a certain antibiotic. 'Why do you think you're allergic to it?' I ask. 'Because when I take it I get an upset stomach,' they reply. 'My doctor said I'm allergic.'

Nine times out of ten this problem is merely an annoying side effect and has nothing to do with an allergic reaction. Nor is such a reaction always unwanted or negative. Antihistamines produce drowsiness, making them unsuitable for children who must remain alert in school. At bedtime the antihistamine's soporific effect can be a blessing, helping children to relax as it relieves their sneezing and itching. Many sedative drugs on the market today actually contain an antihistamine as a primary ingredient.

Side effects can be coped with in several ways, changing the dosage and altering the frequency of administration being the two most common. In some situations nothing can be done to help, and then the medication must simply be changed.

Interactions between drugs When a child takes more than one medication at a time, the possibility always exists that the two will not mix and might produce unexpected and unwanted reactions. It is advisable to check with your child's doctor or local pharmacist regarding the possibility of a reaction when more than one drug is being prescribed.

Coincidental response As part of their natural course, many viral illnesses produce a rash. If a child happens to be taking any medication at the same time, especially an antibiotic, the drug may be accused of causing the rash. In reality, it is a natural response to the virus itself and has nothing to do with the medicine. The problem is that there is no easy way to perform a test and then declare, 'Yes, Johnny's problem is the medication,' or, 'No, the medication had nothing to do with Johnny's rash; the virus caused it.' All a parent can do in this situation is to know that there is a possibility of mistaking one causative factor for another, and to report all suspicious symptoms to the doctor.

Psychogenic reactions I have seen children become dizzy or even pass out after receiving an injection. Almost always this reaction is psychologically triggered, based either on fear of pain or terror of the needle. Rarely, if ever, is it a specific response to the injected material.

Despite the fact that these reactions are psychological rather than physiological, I have heard parents claim that their child experienced a severe allergic reaction while at the doctor's surgery – even after the matter had been thoroughly explained, and seemingly understood. As for the doctor, it is important for him to find out if the child has ever had any previous reactions to injections; if a child is particularly frightened by needles, he should be approached with care. The doctor should explain in clear, simple language what he is going to do and the child should be told what type of examination will be done before the visit. I have found it particularly helpful to illustrate this explanation by giving the first injection (a placebo, of course) to one of the parents. Quite often this example will calm and reassure the child that nothing terrible is going to happen. The time spent in this careful approach will yield dividends in terms of a more co-operative patient and, in general, a better doctor–patient relationship.

IDENTIFYING ALLERGIC DRUG REACTIONS

What type of reaction might one expect if the response is in fact allergic? There are four varieties.

Anaphylactic response This frightening reaction is rapid in onset and simultaneously involves many parts of the body including the skin, lungs, and cardiovascular system. Before it can take place, as with all allergic reactions, previous exposure and sensitization to the offending drug must have occurred. Common symptoms include:

hives

generalized itchy rash

angioedema: swelling of the face involving the lips, tongue, and eyes

nasal discharge, sneezing

shortness of breath, wheezing

drop in blood pressure and rapid heartbeat

The reaction can begin immediately following injection of medication, but more commonly the symptoms occur within thirty to sixty minutes after the drug enters the body.

Cytotoxic response This reaction requires the presence of another class of antibodies, called IgC, in the bloodstream. These antibodies attach to the surface of red blood cells and ultimately lead to their destruction (cytotoxic means 'cell-destroying'). When large numbers of red blood cells are destroyed, a person becomes anaemic. The drugs that can trigger a cytotoxic reaction include the sulpha drugs, various antibiotics and certain anticonvulsant agents. This is not frequent.

Immune complex mediated drug reaction Immune complex reactions occur when large collections of antigens and antibodies are deposited in the skin, blood vessels, kidneys and central nervous system as a result of an allergic response to a drug. The classic example of this phenomenon is a condition called serum sickness, which has the following symptoms:

hives

an itchy, slightly raised rash

swollen, painful joints

tender lymph nodes

fever

This type of allergic response was much more common when vaccines were prepared from horse serum. Today animal serums are rarely used in the manufacture of biological vaccines, and the most common cause of immune complex reactions is penicillin. Serum sickness usually takes from seven to fourteen days to develop. The average duration of symptoms is approximately seven days, but the clinical picture can last for several weeks. Chances for complete recovery are excellent.

Delayed allergic response Contact dermatitis is the most common symptom of a delayed allergic drug reaction. Many drugs applied topically are responsible for causing contact dermatitis. Symptoms can take from three to seven days to develop.

Another variation on this theme is a response to light called a photosensitivity reaction. In some individuals the combination of certain chemical substances (called photoallergens) and exposure to ultraviolet light, from either the sun or an artificial source, causes a photoallergic or a phototoxic rash. The drugs most commonly involved in this reaction include the sulphonamides, griseofulvin (an antifungal drug) and chlorothiazide (a diuretic). Common photoallergens are chemicals found in hair tonics, sunscreens, antiseptic soaps, certain lipstick dyes, and topical antibiotics. The most important method of treating a photosensitivity reaction is avoiding the trouble-causing chemicals.

DIAGNOSING DRUG ALLERGIES

In reviewing the different responses that might result from a drug reaction, it becomes clear that the common allergic symptoms – sneezing, wheezing, and hives – make up only a part of the possible spectrum of reactions. After this review of a list of these potential responses, let's find out how the allergist attempts to evaluate them.

PREPARING FOR THE MEDICAL HISTORY

The starting point is always a detailed medical history. Everything the family and the child can remember about the reaction should be reviewed during the first visit. Because of the limited number of testing procedures available for evaluating drug allergies, this history is especially critical. Things you may wish to tell the doctor include:

> What drug or drugs has the child taken, and in what dose?
>
> What previous exposure, if any, has the child had to the suspected drug or a related class of drugs?
>
> How long after the medicine was given did the symptoms become noticeable?
>
> Describe the symptoms.
>
> How long do the symptoms last?
>
> What treatment, if any, was given? What was the response to treatment?
>
> When the suspected medication was discontinued, what changes, if any, were noted in the child's symptoms? How long did it take for the symptoms to clear up?

TEST PROCEDURES

Once the history and physical examination have been completed, the doctor will then have to decide if he can use the medical laboratory to help him make the diagnosis. Unfortunately there is currently a lack of available specific testing procedures to evaluate most suspected allergic drug reactions. The problem facing research scientists who are trying to develop these testing procedures is that when a drug enters the body many breakdown products are formed. Any one or combination of these biologically active compounds may then be responsible for the suspected allergic reaction. But which ones? That's the question. Putting the pieces of the puzzle into place is a formidable process and so far scientists have been able to accomplish this task for only a small number of medicines. One of the drugs for which a test has been developed is penicillin.

The following list includes those tests which have proved most effective in determining drug sensitivity.

Direct skin tests Direct, in vivo procedures are available for a very limited number of drugs. These include tests for egg-containing vaccines, penicillin, insulin, and tetanus toxoid. A positive response develops within twenty minutes and consists of a raised, itchy wheal at the site of the prick or puncture. (For specific details on direct skin testing, see page 41.)

Patch tests Patch tests are used to determine if a particular drug is causing contact dermatitis. For this test a sample of the drug (antigen) is placed directly on the patient's back or forearm and the test site is covered with an adhesive patch. It is then examined after forty-eight hours. The presence of an irritation with redness and small blisters at the test site is a positive response. This type of test does *not* provide information for symptoms caused by oral medications. (For further information on patch testing, see page 44.)

In vitro or laboratory tests The only in vitro test (i.e. test done in the laboratory) now available for drug sensitivity is the radioallergo-sorbent test (RAST).

The RAST test (see page 41) is currently used for the detection of penicillin allergy; no other drugs can be evaluated with this procedure. Since this test is not performed directly on the patient, it does have the obvious advantage of being risk free.

Challenge test In this test a drug suspected of causing an allergic reaction is administered directly to the patient. If a reaction follows, it proves without question that the child is allergic to the tested drug. Such an approach can of course be highly dangerous and should be attempted only under strict medical supervision. Challenge testing for drugs, on the whole, is rarely indicated.

IDENTIFYING ALLERGIC REACTIONS TO SPECIFIC DRUGS

One basic fact must be stated at the beginning of this section. Solely on the basis of a child's physical signs and symptoms there is no way either you as the parent or I as the doctor can identify the specific cause of an adverse drug reaction. A doctor cannot examine a youngster and then tell the parent which drug is responsible for the symptoms. While certain types of reaction may be more frequently associated with one drug or another, there is no truly consistent pattern when it comes to the confusing world of drug reactions.

PENICILLIN

In the four decades since penicillin was discovered, it has been one of the safest drugs available to doctors. Billions of doses have been prescribed through the years with proportionately few serious side effects. And yet, safe as it is, penicillin is so widely prescribed that it is responsible for the majority of drug-induced anaphylactic deaths.

What symptoms can be caused by an allergic reaction to penicillin? The response may be localized or generalized, a relatively minor inconvenience or a potential catastrophe! The degree of response can range from an itchy contact dermatitis rash to the life-threatening symptoms of anaphylactic shock. (For a discussion of anaphylactic shock, see the chapter on allergic emergencies, page 298.)

At times penicillin reactions will be delayed, occurring from six to eight days after treatment has begun, usually in the form of hives or serum sickness with the following symptoms: fever, rash, swollen lymph nodes, joint swelling, pain and angioedema. Still another reaction occasionally associated with penicillin is haemolytic anaemia, which results from the destruction of red blood cells. Fortunately this condition is very uncommon, and is especially rare in childhood.

By far the most frequent reaction to penicillin is a measles-like rash consisting of small, slightly raised areas found mainly on the arms, legs and trunk. The skin lesions may range in colour from a pale pink to purple. The rash generally clears without specific treatment within fourteen to twenty-one days. The exact cause of this reaction is unknown. It may be toxic and nonallergic. Note, too, that certain penicillin derivates such as Ampicillin will cause a maculopapular rash in 5 to 15 per cent of people. This response is a side effect of the drug, not a true allergic reaction. If your child develops a rash while taking Ampicillin, specific penicillin allergy testing will be necessary. This is the only way to determine whether the rash was a true allergic reaction or merely an unwanted, confusing side effect of this drug.

When penicillin enters the body it is metabolized into a number of breakdown products, the two main components being the major and the minor determinants. An allergic reaction to one or both of these breakdown products is responsible for the clinical symptoms of penicillin sensitivity. Testing should always be done for both major and minor determinants. A positive response to the minor determinant mixture tells the doctor that your child is at risk of developing an anaphylactic reaction from penicillin. A positive reaction to the major determinant indicates that a rapid onset of generalized hives is likely.

The test procedure consists of a series of skin tests using both prick and intradermal techniques. Both the major determinant and the minor determinant mixture are tested first with the prick technique, and if that is negative, intradermal testing is performed. A positive reaction consists of a red, raised, itchy area at the test site which develops within twenty minutes.

What happens if your child tests positively for penicillin allergy but nevertheless must take this drug to cure a life-threatening infection? In such a situation it is possible to desensitize the patient by either an oral or intravenous technique. The patient is started on minute amounts of the drug and the dosage is slowly increased over a period of eight to twelve hours until it reaches a therapeutic dose. This procedure provides immunity on a temporary basis by overwhelming the body's capacity to react allergically only while the child is receiving the drug. When the penicillin is stopped, the sensitivity will return within two or three days. This means that if penicillin must be given again, the complete desensitization process must be repeated. Desensitization programmes must be carried out under direct medical supervision, preferably in a hospital where emergency treatment is available.

There are a few last important points concerning penicillin sensitivity.

Skin testing for penicillin should be done only for patients who are suspected of having had a previous reaction to this drug or a related antibiotic.

Penicillin allergy is not hereditary. The fact that Aunt Rita and cousin Tommy are allergic to Ampicillin does not mean that your child is at an increased risk.

Studies have shown that only 10 to 20 per cent of people who are suspected of having penicillin allergy show a positive response when tested for it. Many people who think they are allergic to penicillin actually tolerate it quite well.

Orally administered penicillin is less prone to cause an allergic reaction than the same drug given intravenously or by injection.

If a skin test is positive, it means there is a very good chance that an allergic reaction will develop if penicillin is taken. If the test is *negative*, this is by no means a guarantee that the patient cannot at some future time become sensitive to this drug.

ASPIRIN (ACETYL SALICYLIC ACID)

As stated above, aspirin and aspirin-containing medications are now contra-indicated in children under twelve. This is a relatively new recommendation and is because of the recognition of the potentially fatal Reye's syndrome, which is associated with taking aspirin. Up until the last year or so aspirin has been one of the main standbys of the family medicine chest useful for all the minor aches and pains of childhood. Luckily there is another product, paracetamol, which is almost as effective, and in the proper dose it is safe. Aspirin is still used for children over twelve and under close medical supervision in conditions where there is no effective substitute, such as Still's disease (children's rheumatoid arthritis).

Aspirin is a potent source of adverse drug reactions. A more accurate term than 'allergy' would be 'idiosyncrasy'. The reaction is a qualitatively abnormal response to the drug, and no definite allergic response patterns have been found.

What should make you suspect that Johnny has a problem with aspirin? By far the most common symptoms caused by a reaction to aspirin is the appearance of hives or angioedema.

There is a condition called the aspirin 'triad' consisting of severe bronchial asthma, sinusitis and nasal polyps. It is found in people with a sensitivity to aspirin. Fortunately, this symptom is almost exclusively a problem for adults.

However, a word of caution. If one of your older children has symptoms of chronic rhinitis and is diagnosed as having nasal polyps, stop using aspirin.

Another group of drugs to avoid are those known as non-steroidal anti-inflammatory drugs (NSAID), which cross-react with aspirin. The first to come on the market was Ibuprofen under the trade name of Brufen as a prescription-only medicine. Recently it has been sold as an over-the-counter medicine under the trade name Nurofen.

Ibuprofen is also prescribed under its own name as a generic drug and under the following trade names: Apsifen, Ebufac, Fenbid, Ibulan, Ibumetin, Motrin and Paxofen.

The most common members of this ever-growing group are:

Naproxen (Naprosyn and Laraflex)

Diflunisal (Dolobid)

Sulindac (Clinoril)

Fenoprofen (Fenapron)

Flurbiprofen (Froben)

Ketoprofen (Alrheumat and Orudis)

Azapropazone (Rheumox)

Mefenamic acid (Ponstan)

Indomethacin (Indocid, Imbrilon, Indoflex, Indolar, Indomad, Mobilan, Rheumacin LA, Slo-Indo)

This group of drugs is used to treat musculoskeletal pains and arthritis symptoms.

Paracetamol is the drug of choice to keep in the medicine cabinet for general family use. It is cheapest at the chemist under its own generic name, but the tablets are rather chalky and difficult to swallow compared with the more palatable forms such as Panadol, Panasorb and Hedex.

Paracetamol comes in liquid form for young children as the generic elixir or mixture and the better-known Calpol or Disprol (which is to be preferred since it is sugar-free and therefore better for the teeth).

Approximately 15 per cent of aspirin-sensitive patients also react to a dye known as tartrazine or E102, see Appendix.

There are no available tests to prove that a person is sensitive to aspirin. A direct challenge test can be done, but as I have stated before this is potentially dangerous and must be carried out only under direct medical supervision.

Finally, in instances where a child has had a reaction to aspirin but where aspirin is absolutely essential for the treatment of a specific medical problem – as in some forms of juvenile rheumatoid arthritis or in rheumatic fever – a method of desensitization is available similar to that used for penicillin (see above). Once desensitization has been carried out, however, aspirin will be tolerated only as long as it is given on a continuous basis and, as with penicillin desensitization, the allergic sensitivity will return when the drug is discontinued.

LOCAL ANAESTHETICS

Adverse reactions to local anaesthetic agents occur most commonly in the dentist's chair, especially after a child has received an injection of a painkiller such as Xylocaine. Reactions can range from mild discomfort to a life-threatening emergency and may stem from toxic responses, psychological causes, or allergic reactions.

Allergic reactions are the least frequent of the three. Ordinarily they consist of a contact sensitivity, an itch or rash. Usually they are caused by a topical over-the-counter cream or ointment, an anti-itch preparation, for instance, or a haemorrhoid salve that contains anaesthetics. Generally speaking, allergic reactions to injected local anaesthetics are very unusual.

Toxic reactions are more frequent. These are due to several possible mechanisms: unknowingly injecting the anaesthetic into a blood vessel, intolerance to a normally absorbed drug or possibly overdosage due to ultra-rapid absorption. Symptoms occur when the medication reaches the central nervous and cardiovascular systems.

The most common story is: Julie went to the dentist and received an injection of a painkiller; then the trouble began. Symptoms may consist of slurred speech, restlessness, dizziness, nausea, vomiting, confusion progressing to convulsions, coma, a drop in blood pressure, cardiac failure and possibly death.

By far the most frequent type of reaction to a topical anaesthetic agent is caused by a vasovagal response. Here just the *thought* of a dental appointment or impending surgery can precipitate dizziness, palpitations and fainting. The condition is, in short, a psychological reaction, one which in many cases can be helped best by discussing the anxiety with your doctor or dentist.

Finally, note that local anaesthetics can be divided into two groups which are chemically quite different from one another. It would be quite unusual for a person to have an allergic reaction to members of both these groups. If a child has a reaction to an anaesthetic from one, the doctor will normally substitute a drug from the second, usually with complete success. If there is a concern that a child has had reactions to both groups of anaesthetic agents, direct skin testing can be performed; however, the results are not absolutely diagnostic.

The amide type of anaesthetic is less likely to give reactions; it includes lignocaine, eupivacaine, and prilocaine. The other type is the ester type which includes amethocaine, benzocaine, cocaine and procaine and most hypersensitivity reactions come from this second group.

X-RAY CONTRAST MEDIA

Today many specialized X-ray studies require the intravenous injection of iodine-containing compounds called radiographic contrast media (RCM). In approximately 5 per cent of patients who are tested, adverse reactions occur within three minutes after the injection of the contrast media. Although extremely unusual, it is possible to develop kidney failure within twenty-four hours of the injection.

It is not clear exactly why these reactions develop. A true allergic mechanism has only rarely been proved and most reactions have been labelled anaphylactoid.

The usual symptoms associated with this response are hives, a drop in blood pressure, angioedema, wheezing and shock. Other findings have included vomiting, nausea, tingling sensations of the arms and legs, and profuse sweating.

Unfortunately, there are deaths associated with these procedures; the statistics approximate the frequency to be somewhat between 1 in 10,000 and 1 in 400,000 patients receiving contrast media injections. However, the vast majority of contrast media reactions are mild and of very short duration.

While there is certainly reason to be absolutely sure that an X-ray study is necessary before going ahead with it, the possibility of an adverse reaction occurring from the RCM is extremely small. And when a reaction to contrast media does take place, children appear to be at far less risk than adults.

At present no foolproof pre-test exists to determine whether a patient will have an adverse reaction to RCM. The best that can be offered is the administration of a small trial dose of the dye immediately before the test begins. If the patient shows no adverse reactions to this sample, then a full dose can be given, *usually* – but not always – safely. Another approach, especially for patients who have had a reaction in the past, involves the administration of both cortisone and the antihistamine Benadryl twenty-four hours before the test is performed, though once again this procedure helps some but not all patients. Fortunately, with the advent of newer imaging techniques such as the CAT scan and Magnetic Resonance Imaging (MRI), the frequency with which contrast media studies are performed will be decreasing, and no doubt there will be a proportional drop in the number of adverse reactions as a result.

INSULIN

While diabetes is certainly not infrequent among children, the majority of adverse insulin responses occur in adults. Reactions to insulin run the gamut from local skin eruptions to generalized anaphylaxis, though just how prevalent these reactions are is difficult to determine. In the medical literature, estimates of insulin sensitivity have ranged from as low as 1 per cent to as high as 50 per cent. Significantly, it is known that approximately one-tenth of all diabetic patients will at some time require changes in their insulin therapy; that's a pretty good indication that insulin sensitivity is not a negligible factor among the diabetic population.

Types of allergic insulin reactions include the following:

Wheal and flare This skin response starts within two to three weeks after insulin therapy is begun. Symptoms consist of local redness (flares) and swelling (wheals) at the injection site. They usually appear fifteen minutes after the dose has been given and then disappear within two to three hours.

Late-phase response Some diabetics develop a wheal and flare response locally, three to six hours after the insulin has been administered. The area involved becomes red and quite painful. It clears within twenty-four hours.

Delayed reaction Delayed reactions appear eight to twelve hours after injection. They are characterized by itchy, well-outlined, painful and slightly swollen areas at the injection site. Discomfort increases hourly, reaching its peak in twenty-four hours. The condition usually takes several days to disappear entirely.

Generalized reaction This response is infrequent but may be quite severe when it occurs. It can include hives, itching, angioedema and shock.

For patients prone to allergic insulin responses, switching from pork to beef insulin or to a more purified variety will often solve the problem. In some cases, insulin desensitization procedures are also appropriate. A diabetes specialist or an allergist can provide you with information regarding these specialized techniques.

PREVENTION, TREATMENT AND CONTROL OF ALLERGIC DRUG REACTIONS

AVOIDANCE

If your child has had some form of adverse reaction to a specific drug, avoidance is by far the best – and often the only – treatment. Problems arise because it is generally impossible to know in advance which drugs will trigger adverse reactions, how these reactions will affect your child and which medicines on the market contain the harmful drug. This is especially true if the drug in question happens to be a common one such as aspirin.

Still, certain steps can be taken:

> Copy down the names of any medicine to which your child has reacted in the past. Do not rely on the doctor to keep these records for you. Even if he has such information on file, he may not always be available when the data is needed. Keep your own records. Carefully update them as required.

> As soon as your child reaches a responsible age, she should be given all pertinent information regarding drugs and/or foods containing the allergenic substance. If parents and child work together on this project, prevention can become a successful family affair.

> Whenever the information is available, familiarize yourself with those drugs that interreact adversely with one another. It is important to know that an aspirin–sensitive asthmatic child should avoid foods and medicines which contain tartrazine dyes. At the same time, with the flood of new medications on the market the subject of cross-reactions among drugs is becoming so complicated that it is virtually impossible to keep track of them all.

When adverse drug reactions do occur, treatment with antihistamines, adrenaline, bronchodilators and, when necessary, cortisone will almost always control symptoms.

Get into the habit of reading the labels on all medicine bottles before giving the medication to your child. If you have any questions about whether a particular offending chemical is contained in these medicines, consult your doctor and/or contact the drug company directly.

If your child is sensitive to a particular drug, it may be wise to have him wear a name tag and keep an identification card in his wallet identifying the specific allergy and/or the problematic drug. Metal wristbands or necklaces identifying the allergy are also useful. While a number of companies market these items, perhaps the best-known is the Medic Alert bracelet, information on which can be obtained from your doctor or from most chemists.

PROVOCATIVE DRUG TESTING

If no test is available to confirm a possible drug sensitivity and it is *absolutely necessary* to use the drug, a challenge test may become necessary. A small dose of the suspect medication is given to the child, who is then closely watched *in* the doctor's surgery for several hours. Such a test is not without some risk, and the decision to perform it must be based both on the severity of the child's original reaction and on the unavailability of a nonrelated drug that would be equally effective in treating the conditon.

DESENSITIZATION

This therapeutic technique has been discussed and described throughout this chapter. Currently it is available for a limited number of drugs including aspirin, penicillin and insulin. The point to be made again here is that desensitization to a drug is *always* temporary and lasts only as long as the child continues to receive the medication. Despite this drawback, however, desensitization does represent the only really satisfactory way we have of safely administering an absolutely necessary drug to a needy allergic patient, and its enormous value should be obvious to everyone.

QUESTIONS AND ANSWERS ABOUT DRUG ALLERGIES

Is there any relationship between drug allergies and the seasons of the year?

No, seasonal patterns do not in any way affect allergic drug responses. A person who is sensitive to a specific medicine in the snows of February will react just as readily to this drug in the heat of July.

What should be done if a child who is reputedly allergic to tetanus toxoid steps on a rusty nail?

In the case of a child with a *proven* allergy to tetanus toxoid, a special tetanus antitoxin can be used. This substance is made from material prepared from human rather than horse serum. It is also possible to do a skin test for tetanus toxoid in advance to check for the possibility of allergy. If the test is negative, the immunization can then be performed without worry. True allergic reactions to tetanus toxoid are extremely rare.

Can a child die from serum sickness?

Serum sickness, a condition that develops following the administration of an animal serum (such as horse serum) or a drug (such as penicillin), rarely if ever ends in death. Still, the symptoms can sometimes be severe. They include fever, hives and painful joints which usually develop anywhere from six to ten days after the medication or animal serum has been administered. The condition usually clears within one to two weeks. Rarely, the symptoms may linger for more than a month.

Can any medicine cause an allergic reaction?

Yes. Certainly some drugs have an especially low allergic risk associated with them. Yet a doctor can never say with absolute assurance that any drug is 100 per cent safe.

Can a drug reaction ever produce permanent effects?

On the whole the chances are exceedingly small. Still, one must never say 'never' when talking about medicine. For instance, there is an unlikely possibility that the blood, bone marrow and neurological system of a child may be affected by certain unusual drug reactions, with resultant organ damage and long-term lingering problems. These cases, however, make up such a tiny percentage of the total number of drug reactions that they are worth mentioning only to keep the record straight.

Is it true that once a child becomes allergic to a drug she will always be allergic to it?

If a child is truly allergic to a medication and does not simply have an idiosyncratic or toxic reaction, chances are that her sensitivity will last. A good general recommendation is to keep the child away from any drugs that have been a proven cause of allergic trouble in the past. It is hoped that in the coming years we will possess an increased number of accurate testing methods for drug allergies. Until then, caution is the rule.

Are drug sensitivities inherited?

There is no evidence to indicate that they are. There may be certain situations in which a specific enzyme is genetically absent from an entire population of people, causing this group to be incapable of tolerating a specific drug. An example is the prima-quine-induced haemolytic anaemia found in people deficient in the enzyme glucose 6-phosphate dehydrogenase. Given normal circumstances, allergies to common drugs such as aspirin or penicillin are not inherited.

CHAPTER ELEVEN

Allergic Skin Conditions

An allergist is often called upon to see children with a variety of skin rashes suspected of 'being caused by an allergy'. The most frequent dermatological problem I have encountered in my practice is a form of eczema called atopic dermatitis. Other frequently seen rashes belong to the category of contact dermatitis, which has many possible causes. In this chapter I will concentrate on atopic and contact dermatitis and touch only briefly on other skin conditions.

ECZEMA

Susan, aged three, was carried into my office in her mother's arms. Unable to extend her arms and legs, she kept them tightly flexed close to her body. Her fingers were clenched into fists and the skin on her face was as red and rough as the skin of a sailor. Her mother smiled sadly. 'Eczema,' she said, 'and today is one of her better days.'

Adam was six years old when he first came to see me. He sat in the chair opposite mine. During the entire visit he proceeded to itch, dig and literally tear at the irritating skin eruptions covering a good part of his little body. 'He's always like this,' his mother informed me. 'It never stops!'

Jane was only two years old when her mother brought her to my office. Jane's doctor had noticed a small reddish patch on her cheeks some weeks earlier. He sent her to me for a diagnosis. By the time Jane arrived, the patch had almost doubled in size. 'I tried to stop her from scratching it,' both parents told me, 'but short of putting her into a straitjacket there was just nothing we could do!'

Three different children, three different variations on the same theme. It's called eczema. And while it is not a life-threatening menace, it can be one of the most agonizing ailments imaginable. What is it exactly?

Technically speaking, eczema is not a disease at all but a reactive response of the skin. When it is restricted to a single area of the body – usually in the form of small, well-outlined, coin-sized patches that break down easily when scratched, ooze, then finally crust over – the condition is known as nummular eczema. When the eczematous rash spreads across the body and forms larger, thickened, purplish-red lesions over sheetlike areas, as it frequently does, it becomes generalized eczema. The rash is characteristically found in the bends of the elbows, on the neck and face, behind the ears, and at the backs of the knees. The appearance of the skin itself may change considerably during the various stages of the disorder: acute, chronic and subacute.

Acute stage. Characterized by redness, swelling and, when the skin has been broken, a wet, watery look called 'weeping'. These open skin surfaces provide an excellent breeding ground for bacteria and the development of infection. This occurs quite frequently.

Chronic stage. In its more advanced stages, after the weeping has dried, the rash takes on a dry, dark, thickened, scaling and leathery appearance.

Subacute stage. Includes characteristics of both the acute and chronic.

ATOPIC DERMATITIS

Atopic dermatitis is the most common form of childhood eczema. It strikes approximately 1 to 3 per cent of all infants during their first two years of life and continues to lurk as a threat for youngsters of all ages into the teenage years. Among eczema sufferers a strong family history of allergy is quite common – eczema is most likely hereditary – and figures show that a sizeable percentage of atopic dermatitis patients have other allergies. Approximately 40 to 50 per cent of children with atopic dermatitis develop hay fever, and between 15 and 30 per cent are asthmatic. The good news is that roughly half of atopic dermatitis sufferers will spontaneously lose their eczema before becoming adults, and a majority of the remaining percentage have an excellent chance of controlling their condition.

HOW TO IDENTIFY ATOPIC DERMATITIS

Although most allergists agree that atopic dermatitis is an allergic condition, it is usually quite difficult to pinpoint the specific causes of the problem. Certainly for a significant number of children foods play a role, either as a primary triggering agent or as a secondary aggravating factor. By both clinical observation and the use of such procedures as the prick skin tests (see page 41) or the RAST test (see page 41), it is occasionally possible to prove that a specific food sensitivity is responsible for the atopic dermatitis. Unfortunately, this does not happen too often. In fact, much to the doctor's chagrin and frustration, atopic dermatitis is most often brought under control entirely *without* knowledge on his part of what actually caused it.

So strong is the itch associated with atopic dermatitis in some young patients that several decades ago it was not unusual to walk into the children's ward of a hospital and see infants with severe eczema with their arms and legs loosely held in restraints, the theory being that if the patients were kept from scratching their skin, the rash would subside. Because of the potentially harmful psychological effects which could develop from this treatment, it was finally abandoned. Still, the point was well made, and should be well made here: there is no doubt that if scratching is prevented in a child suffering from atopic dermatitis, even the worst eczematous rash can often be made to disappear completely. A prominent dermatologist stated that with atopic dermatitis, 'It isn't the eruption that itches but the itch that erupts.' The moral is that if you control the itch, you control the rash.

Atopic dermatitis can be identified by its red lesions, dry skin and intense itching. The primary task of both parents and doctors when faced with the taxing problem of the child with atopic dermatitis is to monitor all symptoms closely and get appropriate treatment as soon as possible. I will detail below some of the specific methods by which these tasks can be accomplished.

THE STAGES OF ATOPIC DERMATITIS

Infantine stage – up to two years of age Though clinical symptoms of atopic dermatitis almost never appear before the age of one month, the majority of children develop their symptoms during the first year of life. Once the rash has become apparent, certain environmental conditions can aggravate the situation immensely. Winter – with its dry, cold air, heavy, irritating clothing and reduction of direct skin exposure to sunlight – is a particularly rough time for most eczema sufferers. Symptoms also seem to intensify when a youngster has a mild cold, is teething or is going through a stressful period. Curiously, some children with atopic dermatitis usually experience a *decrease* in rash symptoms when suffering from measles or other viral illness. We are not sure why this is so.

The earliest signs of atopic dermatitis usually appear on the face, especially on the cheeks, in the form of a patchy red rash. If this mild eruption is not vigorously treated, it can spread with shocking speed. I have seen a number of cases in which a small outbreak begins innocently enough on the face and then proceeds to spread over most of the body in less than a month. This type of generalized spreading can become so severe that it makes the child who was previously an angel and a delight turn into a weeping, restless, miserable waif who finds neither an hour's relief nor a moment's peace.

Not every child, of course, develops widespread rashes. I have seen many instances where only the cheeks are involved; interestingly enough, the nose and area around the mouth almost always seem to be spared. In addition to lesions on the cheeks, eczema frequently involves the backs of the ears, producing deep cracks that ooze and bleed. Other affected areas include the neck, scalp, arms, sides of the legs and the ankles. Regardless of where the rash is located, I can't recall ever seeing a patient with atopic dermatitis who didn't have severe itching. A cardinal rule to bear in mind: if the rash does not itch, it isn't atopic dermatitis.

Childhood stage – from age two to twelve Children with eczema between the ages of two and twelve usually have very dry skin with localized lesions that tend to form in the creases and the flexed parts of the arms, neck and legs. The skin behind the ears is another commonly involved area.

Because of the persistent itch and chronic scratching associated with eczema, the skin tends to become tough and thickened with an almost leathery consistency that is rough to the touch (skin in this condition is described as being lichenified). Children whose eczema persists into the school years quite often appear unhappy, withdrawn and antisocial. Because of the seeming hopelessness of their condition and the embarrassment of unsightly skin, such children frequently become loners and self-imposed exiles. In school they may be difficult to manage, constantly at odds with teacher and pupils alike, while at home they find it difficult to get along with other family members. These young people need all the assurance and support they can get from everyone in their vicinity: parents, siblings, friends, teachers and doctor.

It is not unusual for school-age children who developed their atopic dermatitis during infancy to 'outgrow' their skin symptoms. That's the good news. The bad news is that a sizeable number of these youngsters will go on to develop hay fever and/or asthma symptoms.

Adolescent and adult stage By the time a youngster has reached adolescence, quite often the eczema of the early childhood years has disappeared. If it has continued into the teenage years or begins at this time of life, the skin lesions tend to be of the dry, lichenified variety. The rash will mainly be found on the inside surface of the arms and legs as well as the wrists and hands. A rash present at this time will probably continue to some extent into the adult years.

THE ROLE OF FOODS IN ATOPIC DERMATITIS

Many studies suggest that during the first six months of life, avoidance of potentially allergenic foods such as milk, eggs and wheat is helpful in retarding the development of atopic dermatitis.

Of these foods, milk is by far the most likely to cause trouble. At the onset of symptoms, try replacing it with a non-dairy formula. Soybean preparations such as Wysoy and Isomil or non-dairy preparations such as meat-based or lamb-based formulas are all possible substitutes. Breastfeeding, an increasing trend, is believed to help in decreasing the risk of developing allergy conditions, especially in children with a hereditary predisposition.

While it is often difficult to pinpoint the specific foods that cause trouble, there is no question that food allergy plays a definite role in atopic dermatitis. If you have any suspicions in this direction, it would be wise to use a milk substitute and eliminate all suspected foods from the diet. Dietary regulation is one of the most important methods we have for both determining the cause and treating the symptoms of atopic dermatitis. Before making any major changes in your child's diet, however, always speak to your doctor. A well-balanced diet must be the foundation of any nutritional programme.

DISTINGUISHING ATOPIC DERMATITIS FROM OTHER SKIN DISORDERS

A number of skin conditions cause a rash that may be confused with atopic dermatitis. A brief description of these look-alikes follows.

Seborrhoeic dermatitis The table opposite will provide you with a comparison of these two common skin problems of early infancy.

Nappy rash This frequently irritating, itchy rash is limited exclusively to the nappy area. It is a result of a yeast or fungus infection or an irritation from ammonia, a normal component of urine. This condition responds quite well to appropriate topical treatment and frequent nappy changes.

Contact dermatitis While it is true that there is a great deal of itching associated with contact dermatitis, the rash is usually localized to one area of the body. Treatment with a cortisone-containing cream or ointment usually eliminates the problem. The condition is caused by sensitivity to a variety of chemicals ranging from plants

Table 11 Identifying atopic dermatitis

	Seborrhoeic dermatitis	Atopic dermatitis
Type of rash	Salmon-coloured Greasy scales Clearly outlined	Reddened, localized in single dry patches or generalized. Rash is often weeping and bloody because of constant scratching
Distribution of rash	Begins in scalp and progresses downwards. Facial involvement is usually partial. Found on neck, under the arms, on lower abdomen and genital regions	Found commonly on the face, mainly the cheeks. The neck, sometimes the scalp, the arms, legs and trunk
Itch	Rarely present	Most important symptom
Onset	Usually within the first two months of life	Generally after the age of two months
Family history of allergy	Usually absent	Usually present

such as primulas to penicillin. Unlike atopic dermatitis, the rash is produced *exclusively* by sensitivity to things outside the body.

Tinea dermatitis This is caused by a variety of different fungal agents. The lesions can in some situations be confused with atopic dermatitis. The best-known form is tinea pedis, commonly called athlete's foot. Other examples are tinea capitis, ringworm of the scalp, and tinea circinata, ringworm involving the face, neck and arms.

The rash caused by this fungus is usually a solitary, circular lesion with sharply outlined borders. On the scalp the lesion will produce a circumscribed local area of hair loss. The specific diagnosis is made by looking at scrapings from the lesions under a microscope. There are effective oral and topical medicines for this condition.

Pityriasis rosea The typical appearance of pityriasis consists of slightly raised, salmon-coloured lesions on the trunk. The rash can vary in shade from pale yellow to light red. The condition usually begins with a small round lesion on the chest or back called the herald patch. Unlike atopic dermatitis, pityriasis rarely has any associated itching. It is self-limiting, which means that it will clear up by itself within four to eight weeks.

POSSIBLE COMPLICATIONS OF ATOPIC DERMATITIS

Perhaps surprisingly, there are two rare but potentially life-threatening complications that can occur in a child with atopic dermatitis. One of them, eczema vaccinatum, has become considerably less of a problem since routine smallpox vaccinations have been discontinued. In brief, contact with smallpox vaccine or with individuals who have been vaccinated can produce smallpox-like lesions in a child with atopic dermatitis. Any person with atopic dermatitis should *never* be exposed to anyone who has recently been vaccinated for smallpox.

The other potentially severe condition is called either eczema herpeticum or Kaposi's varicelliform eruption. Exposure to and infection with the virus herpes simplex, which is responsible for cold sores, is the cause of the problem. The rash that develops looks like chicken pox and is found mainly on the face and those parts of the body where atopic dermatitis is active.

If there are large open skin areas which are weeping, then secondary bacterial infection and major problems caused by the loss of fluids and essential minerals can develop. A child with this condition may require admission to the hospital for supportive therapy.

Today I can still remember an eight-year-old boy named Carl who had chronic atopic dermatitis. For several hours one afternoon he had been in close contact with a friend who had several cold sores on his lip. Within a few days Carl was admitted to hospital with severe eczema herpeticum. For seventy-two hours his temperature ranged between 104 and 106 degrees, and despite the latest in cooling techniques, antipyretic drugs and round-the-clock nursing, we were unable to break the fever. Finally, on the fourth hospital day, as I was becoming convinced the boy would surely die, his fever began to fall and his skin lesions started to dry. From then on his recovery was slow but regular. Today, it might be added, at twenty-three, Carl is a six-foot-three giant, with, among many other personal assets, perfect skin. Even in the worst of medical situations, a positive outcome is possible.

Lesser but still significant complications can also result. Children with atopic dermatitis are at increased risk of developing superficial staph and strep skin infections. Such problems must be carefully watched for and aggressively treated with appropriate antibiotics if they appear. Any child with atopic dermatitis who begins complaining of difficulty in seeing or blurred vision must be examined by an eye specialist for the possible presence of atopic cataracts. This is a very rare complication involving the lens of the eye that can have a harmful effect on a child's vision. A brief examination can determine whether a cataract is present.

One possible cause for this problem may be the prolonged use of oral cortisone drugs. Any child who must take this medicine for a long time should be checked at least once a year by an ophthalmologist.

LABORATORY EVALUATION

As a rule, the diagnosis of atopic dermatitis is made on the basis of a complete history and a thorough physical examination. The laboratory, unfortunately, can provide your doctor with relatively little assistance when it comes to this condition.

The IgE level, which is selectively elevated in allergic patients, is abnormally high in almost 100 per cent of children with atopic dermatitis.

Most children with atopic dermatitis have highly irritable skin and are therefore poor candidates for direct allergy skin tests. I have also not been very impressed with the information obtained from skin testing. On rare occasions a RAST test has been helpful in pinpointing specific causes for a child's eczema.

In the final analysis, perhaps the most effective testing and treatment approach to eczema is simply environmental control. Eliminate from your home substances that tend to cause allergic symptoms such as wool, feathers, dust and animal dander. For the younger child, dietary manipulation with the removal and reintroduction of certain groups of foods can be especially helpful (see the chapter on food allergies for more details about diet control).

A four-month-old named Robert was brought to my consulting room with a suspicious-looking rash on his cheeks and ears. Robert had been placed on a milk-based formula on which he had thrived since birth. I ordered the formula suspended for ten days and substituted a soy-based preparation. Within the week the rash entirely disappeared. We next reintroduced the milk formula to Robert's diet and the rash quickly returned. The soy-based formula was then tried again, with the same positive results, and the family was convinced. Milk was removed from Robert's diet for the next six months and he remained free of the rash. When milk was reintroduced into his diet, Robert had no skin problems of any kind; his sensitivity had entirely disappeared.

This same method of dietary manipulation can be used with older atopic dermatitis children by removing a specific food or food group from the diet and observing the results. To date this technique is the most effective we have of establishing a causal relationship between specific foods and atopic dermatitis.

HOME CARE FOR A CHILD WITH ATOPIC DERMATITIS

General measures

There are a number of useful things parents can do to decrease and control the symptoms of atopic dermatitis.

When indoor air is dry, use a humidifier to increase the relative humidity to 40 to 45 per cent. The increased moisture in the air will decrease skin irritation and itchiness, especially during the winter when the household atmosphere tends to be dry. While there are many types of humidifiers on the market, an ultrasonic cool mist humidifier in my opinion is the best. More on this below.

Children with eczema should avoid direct contact with obvious allergens, especially wool, feathers, furs and animal dander.

Certain foods with a high potential for causing allergic symptoms – such as milk, eggs and wheat – should be removed for a trial period from the diet of eczematous children. Whatever beneficial changes are going to take place should be evident after seven to fourteen days of avoidance.

Since emotional stress may intensify symptoms of atopic dermatitis, keep the child on an even keel and guide him away from particularly stressful situations. I realize it is easier in today's rather complicated world to make this recommendation than to carry it out, but even small efforts sometimes yield big results. Give it a try.

Control of itching This is probably the single most important management area in the treatment of a child with atopic dermatitis. If the itch–scratch–itch–scratch cycle is interrupted, the skin lesions will tend to heal on their own. Unfortunately there is no uniformly effective anti-itch medication on the market today, and what works for one child fails with another. The drugs which have the best track records in my experience include the following:

> *Phenergan.* This is a well-known antishistamine which is slightly sedative, which it needs to be if it is to have any useful anti-itch properties. It is particularly useful at bedtime, when its sedative properties are particularly desirable, but if used in a lower dose it can be given during the day as well.

> *Vallergan.* This is a similar drug which is perhaps slightly more sedative.

> *Atarax.* This is one of the most effective antihistamines for the control of itching. The starting dose usually is 1 milligram per pound of body weight a day. The dose may be increased every three to four days until the itch abates.

> *Periactin.* For some children this is quite effective. The dose is 0.1 milligram per pound of body weight a day divided in two or three doses.

Effective as antihistamines are when taken orally, these drugs should *never* be applied directly to the skin in a topical preparation; they can sensitize the skin and produce contact dermatitis.

Keep the skin moist In addition to using antihistamines for the control of itching, local skin care measures play a significant role in the overall management of atopic dermatitis. Well-moistened skin is less likely to itch.

The main purpose of skin moistener/lubricant preparations is to retain water within the superficial layers of the skin. One of the least expensive and most accessible of these lubricants is vegetable cooking fats. The problem, of course, with using preparations such as Spry is their greasy feeling, but if they can be tolerated these products are effective lubricants.

Some moisturizers, lubricants or emollients, whether available by prescription or over the counter, contain chemicals which may be irritating rather than soothing for some patients. Examples include paraben, a potential cause of contact dermatitis, and lanolin, a possible problem for children with a strong allergy to wool (lanolin is derived from sheep). Table 12 lists the frequently prescribed lubricants.

Humidification As mentioned above, when the air in a room lacks adequate moisture it causes the skin to become dry and increases its potential for itching. The addition of water vapour to the household atmosphere via electronic humidifiers or by placing pans of water near the heat source in different rooms is a simple and effective way of approaching the situation. In order of increasing efficiency, the following methods will all improve the relative humidity level in your home.

Place pans of water near various heat sources throughout your home, near the radiators, steam pipes, stove.

Set up a cool air vapour humidifier in the child's room and, if possible, in other rooms of the house.

Purchase an ultrasonic cool mist humidifier. Available at most appliance stores, this marvellous machine employs sound waves to break up water into a very fine vapour. The particles released by the mechanism then remain suspended in the air instead of condensing into pockets of moisture on the walls, furniture and floors, as happens with many cool air vapour humidifiers.

The major problem with ultrasonic mist humidifiers is their rather high cost – prices can range from £40 to £100. Since the demand for these useful appliances is steadily increasing, it is likely

Table 12 Moisturizing Preparations

Emulsifying ointment is made from emulsifying wax, white soft paraffin and liquid paraffin or an improved formula is: emulsifying wax, isopropyl myristate, white soft paraffin and liquid paraffin.

Aqueous cream contains emulsifying ointment, chloro-cresol and water.

E 45 cream contains light liquid paraffin, white soft paraffin, wool fat, methyl hydroxybenzoate, self-emulsifying monostearin, stearic acid and triethanolamine.

Alcoderm water-miscible, contains carbomen, cetyl alcohol, liquid paraffin, polysorbate 60, sodium lauryl sulphate, stearyl alcohol, triethanolamine. Additives: isopropyl palminate, hydroxybenzate (parabens).

Emulsiderm liquid emulsion (= lotion) contains liquid paraffin, isopropyl myristate, benzalkonium chloride. Additives: polysorbate 60.

Keri contains mineral oil, lanolin oil. Additives/hydroxybenzoates (parabens), propyline glycol, fragrance.

Oilatum cream contains arachis oil, providone in a water-miscible base.

Aquadrate cream contains urea 10% in a powder in cream base.

Calmurid cream contains urea 10% in lactic acid in a water-miscible base.

---

that competition will soon bring their cost within the reach of most pockets. Look for them in the off-season – at the end of winter – for the best buys.

Finally, the optimal relative humidity level for comfort is in the range of 40 to 45 per cent. A household device called a humidistat will record this figure in much the same way a thermometer tells the room temperature, and it is well worth acquiring. Regardless of the method used to control the water content indoors, however, relative humidity must always be kept at an optimum level without major fluctuations. If carefully monitored, this can save your child many hours of discomfort.

General skin care measures

Bathing The question of whether taking a bath or shower is harmful or beneficial for eczematous patients is much debated. My own feeling is that during the colder months of the year, when children with eczema seem to be most uncomfortable, they should be bathed briefly three or four times a week. Be sure to keep the water in these baths lukewarm, for as the water temperature rises it causes the superficial blood vessels to dilate or open and the surface temperature of the skin to increase, adding to the likelihood of increased itching. The use of bath oils such as Alpha-Keri will also help by retaining moisture within the superficial layers of the skin. Another commercial product with a similar effect is Aveeno, a natural oatmeal derivative that soothes and cleanses the skin.

The simpler the soap, the less likely it is to cause trouble. Chemists sell a simple soap without any deodorants or perfumes which is ideal. Emulsifying ointment may be used as a soap substitute for children who cannot tolerate even the simple soaps.

Most chemists stock special hypoallergenic soaps with a pH level balanced for allergic children. Consult your doctor for the one best suited to your child's condition. In general, use as little soap as possible on the child with atopic dermatitis and give baths only when they are absolutely necessary.

Indoor temperature The temperature in your home should be kept between 20 and 22 degrees Centigrade (68 and 70 degrees Fahrenheit). This is warm enough to keep children comfortable but not so hot that it makes them sweat (as mentioned previously, sweating aggravates skin irritation, which causes increased itching). During the summer, electric fans can be used to maintain household temperatures at a comfortable level.

Nail care One sharp or jagged fingernail can destroy days of a careful skin care regimen. Always keep nails short. When you trim, I suggest you avoid scissors or nail clippers that often leave small sharp edges. An emery board or nail file will get the job done and will provide perfectly smooth nails. Once a day, quickly look at your child's fingernails. The old saying about an ounce of prevention is very appropriate in this situation. When it is practical, the use of cotton gloves on your child's hands at bedtime may limit the damage from nocturnal scratching.

Type of clothing Loose-weave cottons are your best bet. In contact with the skin, these garments are very comfortable. Wool and various synthetic fibres are potentially irritating and should be avoided. Does this mean your child cannot wear a warm woollen winter coat when the thermometer plummets? Most of the time woollen outer garments are pefectly all right, and a cotton scarf worn around the neck will eliminate irritation caused by wool collars. As a rule of thumb, a child who has atopic dermatitis should wear clothing that is loose and comfortable, allowing plenty of circulation with a minimum of binding.

MEDICAL CARE

Several drugs are currently available for treating children with atopic dermatitis:

Topical cortisone For many years cortisone creams, ointments and lotions have been the most important drugs used for the treatment of eczematous skin conditions. If a rash is scaly, dry and itchy, it will probably respond very well to these powerful anti-inflammatory preparations. Of course any time a steroid drug is prescribed, the doctor must consider the possible undesirable side effects. Fortunately, when it comes to topical forms of cortisone the potential dangers are extremely small. You would literally have to dip your child into a vat of cortisone cream several times a day for many weeks before severe side effects would develop.

Apply topical steroids only to those skin areas with a visible rash. Depending on the appearance of the rash, your doctor will prescribe the appropriate form of topical steroid.

Small amounts of topical steroids should be applied to the rash three to four times a day. When the skin begins to clear, the frequency can be decreased and use of the drug eventually discontinued. One very important rule for parents to follow in the treatment of atopic dermatitis is to be aggressive, not to let the rash get ahead of you: it is always harder to catch up than to stay ahead. Even when the rash is under control and the steroid agents are discontinued, always be ready to treat any recurrence vigorously. A list of commonly used steroid preparations is found in Table 13.

One word of caution: eczematous areas on the face should be treated with only the mildest forms of cortisone; the more potent steroid compounds can cause thinning of the skin and acne. While hydrocortisone in a concentration of 0.5 or 1 per cent is particularly appropriate in this case, your doctor should be your ultimate guide for dose and prescription.

What about orally administered steroids? The use of these

Table 13 Topical Steroid Preparations

Generic name	Brand name
Mildly potent	
Hydrocortisone 0.1%	Dioderm cream
Hydrocortisone 0.125%	Dome Cort cream
Hydrocortisone 0.5%	Efcortelan cream, ointment & lotion Cobadex cream
Hydrocortisone 1.0%	Efcortelan cream, ointment & lotion Cobadex cream Hydrocortistab cream & ointment Hydrocortisyl cream & ointment
Hydrocortisone 2.5%	Efcortelan cream & ointment
(Also sold under generic name at various strengths.)	
Alchometasone dipropionate 0.05%	Modrasone cream & ointment
Fluocinolone acetonide 0.0025%	Synalar 1:10
Moderately Potent	
Clobetasone butyrate 0.05%	Eumovate cream & ointment
Desoxymethasone 0.05%	Stiedex LP oily cream
Fluocinolone acetonide 0.00625%	Synalar 1:4 cream & ointment
Fluocortolone hexanoate 0.1% Fluocortolone privalata 0.1%	Ultradil cream & ointment
Fluocortolone 0.25% Fluocortolone hexanoate 0.25%	Ultralanum plain cream & ointment
Flurandrenolone 0.0125%	Haelan cream & ointment
Flurandrenolone 0.05%	Haelan X cream & ointment
Potent	
Beclomethasone dipropionate 0.025%	Propaderm cream & ointment
Betamethasone dipropionate 0.05%	Diprosone cream & ointment
Betamethasone valerate 0.025%	Betnovate RD cream & ointment
Betamethasone valerate 0.1%	Betnovate cream, ointment, lotion & scalp application
Desonide 0.05%	Tridesilon cream & ointment
Desoxymethasone 0.25%	Stiedex oily cream

Generic name	Brand name
	Potent (continued)
Diflucortolone valerate 0.1%	Nerisone cream, oily cream & ointment
	Temetex cream, ointment & fatty ointment
Fluclorone acetonide 0.025%	Topilar cream
Fluocinolone acetonide 0.025%	Synalar cream & ointment
Fluocinonide 0.05%	Metosyn cream & ointment
Hydrocortisone butyrate 0.1%	Locoid cream & ointment
Triamcinolone acetonide 0.1%	Adcortyl cream & ointment
	Ledercort cream & ointment
	Very Potent
Clobetasol propionate 0.05%	Dermovate cream & ointment
Diflucortolone valerate 0.3%	Nerisone Forte oily cream & ointment
Halcinonide 0.1%	Halciderm cream

drugs is usually recommended only if the atopic dermatitis cannot be controlled by any other measure: antihistamine use, diet regulation and/or application of topical steroid agents. Once again, a word of caution: the results of orally administered cortisone are dramatic and the drugs are highly effective, but problems arise over how long the medicine should be given. If the drug is administered for a short time and then discontinued abruptly, most patients will experience a rapid relapse and may be worse off than before the cortisone was taken; the dosage *must* be tapered off slowly. If, on the other hand, the medication is given for long periods of time, unwanted and sometimes dangerous side effects may occur. For these reasons the long-term use of oral steroids for atopic dermatitis should *rarely if ever* be prescribed.

Compresses For acute symptoms of atopic dermatitis, especially lesions that are oozing and wet, compresses will soothe the irritation and dry the rash. These compresses can be made from cool water or Burrow's solution (aluminium acetate).

Compresses are quite effective for cleaning the rash and decreasing local itching. They cause fluids to evaporate and hence cool the wound, making it decidedly more comfortable for the child. Make a compress and apply it directly to the rash for ten to fifteen minutes, two to four times a day. When the acute symptoms have cleared, discontinue treatment.

Antibiotics Quite frequently children with atopic dermatitis develop bacterial skin infections. You as parents must realize that this complication can occur and must be treated promptly with appropriate antibiotics. These infections develop most often on the arms and legs. The first indication of the presence of an infection is enlarged and sensitive lymph glands under the arms or in the groin. Any areas that are draining or appear to be very red are almost certainly infected. This complication develops because the skin surface has been broken by your child's prolonged scratching. Bacteria that are harmless on intact skin are able to get past the protective outer surface of the skin and cause an infection within the deeper layers.

Once the infection has been controlled, the eczematous rash will respond to treatment with topical steroids, lubricants and oral antihistamines. Parents should never use an antibiotic without first consulting a doctor.

Immunotherapy In my opinion, 'allergy jabs' are ineffective for the treatment of a child whose only 'allergic' problem is atopic dermatitis. There certainly are youngsters who have allergic rhinitis or pollen asthma in addition to eczema. In this situation, immunotherapy would be indicated as treatment for the nasal and chest conditions. However, with the present restrictions on immunotherapy, it is not a practical form of therapy for these conditions.

Diet If you are suspicious that a specific food or food family is causing your child's rash, eliminate the suspected offender for two weeks and see if the rash improves. If you are certain that positive changes have taken place, then that food should be eliminated from the diet for a three-to-six-month period. Cautious reintroduction of the food can then be tried to determine if the sensitivity still exists. In some cases the problem will be entirely gone and the child can return to her usual eating pattern.

Whether to perform allergy food tests remains an unanswered

question. Some allergists claim that food testing is very important in the evaluation of a child with atopic dermatitis. In general, I have not found that these tests have helped me in the management of these youngsters. I still rely very heavily on an accurate, detailed food history and elimination diets in attempting to determine if specific foods are playing a role in a child's atopic dermatitis.

CONTACT DERMATITIS

As the name implies, contact dermatitis is typified by skin eruptions resulting from direct contact with a variety of substances, most commonly household products, chemical compounds and plant materials. The rash begins at the point of direct contact and in general tends to remain localized. However, if exposure to the causative agent is repeated, there is a very good chance that the rash will spread. Unlike atopic dermatitis, a contact sensitivity is caused only by substances *external* to the body.

The condition appears in three main forms: allergic contact dermatitis, irritant contact dermatitis and photoallergic contact dermatitis.

Allergic contact dermatitis Children develop this condition after being exposed to a specific chemical, becoming sensitized to it, and developing a rash on subsequent exposure. The resulting dermatitis may be swollen, reddened, blistery or scaly. Itching is a constant symptom. An extremely common example is the rash produced by primulas. Other causes might include hair dyes and, rarely, a sensitivity to airborne allergens.

Irritant contact dermatitis Here the substance causing the dermatitis is either a potent irritant such as a strong acid or a chemical substance. Nappy rash in infants, caused by metabolic breakdown substances in the stool and urine, is a classic example. People who frequently wash their hands with harsh soaps and detergents or those who come into continual contact with commercial chemicals such as cleaning fluids and paints are likewise prime candidates for this form of eczema.

Photoallergic contact dermatitis Two ingredients are essential to produce this condition: a specific chemical sensitizer and exposure to ultraviolet light. Neither alone will produce the rash; only their interaction will set the reaction in motion. As a rule, patients with photoallergic sensitivity are urged to stay out of the sun and to use sunscreen agents. Photoallergic contact dermatitis is the rarest form of contact dermatitis, especially among children.

CAUSES OF CONTACT DERMATITIS

Many of the ordinary chemical compounds used every day can cause contact dermatitis. A definitive list would take up pages. Some representative examples include:

antibiotic creams	leather products
antiperspirants	nail polish
baby oils	paints
bubble bath	perfumes
chromium salts	rubber products
cosmetics	shampoos
fabric dyes	soap
glues	solvents
hair dyes	synthetic fabrics
insecticides	topical anaesthetics
jewellery	turpentine

It is, of course, virtually impossible to escape from all the potentially allergenic chemicals that have become so integral a part of our daily lives, and both parents and children can drive themselves mad by attempting such a thing. On the other hand, ordinary observation and common sense will take one a long way.

For instance, clues to the possible cause of contact dermatitis can be derived by noting the parts of the child's body where the dermatitis is located. If a child develops a rash on her neck, suspicion should be focused on her jewellery; metals in contact with the skin are a frequent cause of contact dermatitis. An outbreak on the wrist may be traced to a watchband or bracelet, and so on. By careful observation, you may be able to identify the substance or substances responsible for the problem.

EVALUATION AND TREATMENT OF ALLERGIC CONTACT DERMATITIS

Evaluation As in all allergic conditions, a detailed history and thorough examination are essential steps in the evaluation of any patient with contact dermatitis. If the doctor suspects that the dermatitis is of the allergic variety, he may then recommend patch testing to determine which substances are causing the problem (see page 44).

Patch testing will be performed after the acute outbreak has been brought under control by appropriate treatment. The patch itself is composed of a soft cloth or paper impregnated with a specific allergen and placed on the upper arm or upper portion of the back. An adhesive bandage-type dressing is fitted over it and the patch area is allowed to incubate for forty-eight hours. (If intense local itching appears before this time, it indicates a high degree of sensitivity. The doctor should be notified right away and the test discontinued.)

Once the forty-eight hours have passed, the patches are removed. The test sites are examined within two to four hours and then examined again two days later. A positive reaction consists of redness, local swelling and blisters at the test site. Once the positive substances are identified, avoiding them will usually prevent recurrence of the rash.

Treatment The rash caused by contact dermatitis is treated in much the same manner as atopic dermatitis. Cool compresses are useful for soothing a weeping rash, and topical steroid creams or ointments will keep most lesions under control. Occasionally, appropriate short doses of oral cortisone will be given for particularly stubborn or severe cases. The skin care and itch control procedures mentioned earlier for atopic dermatitis are equally appropriate for the control of contact dermatitis.

Fortunately, most cases of contact dermatitis can be diagnosed and subsequently treated. Avoidance of the substance responsible for the problem will 'cure' the condition. Permanent skin changes rarely result from contact dermatitis.

QUESTIONS AND ANSWERS ABOUT ECZEMA

Is aspirin ever used to control severe itching associated with atopic dermatitis?

Remember that aspirin should not be given to children under twelve. But there is clinical evidence that some children respond well to aspirin for the control of persistent itching. If you cannot relieve the child's itching with antihistamines, then aspirin is worth a try for an older child.

What effect, if any, does being outdoors in sunny weather have on a child's atopic dermatitis?

During the warmer months of the year many children with atopic dermatitis tend to benefit from being outdoors. Exposure to sunlight decreases the intensity of eczematous rashes, and for some children the sun appears to have an almost miraculous effect; their skin becomes less dry and itching decreases dramatically. The seaside is especially therapeutic, and for the majority of young sufferers the blend of salt water and sunlight has a wonderfully healing influence.

Is eczema ever contagious?

Though the characteristic rash it produces certainly has a menacing appearance, eczema is in no way contagious and one child cannot under any circumstances 'catch' it from another. The only time contagion becomes an issue is when a secondary infection accompanies the eczema, and even then it is the infection that spreads, not the atopic dermatitis.

Once eczema has disappeared, will the child continue to have dry skin into adult life?

The tendency to a dry skin is something you are usually born with. I would say that your particular skin characteristics, whether oily or dry, persist through life.

What happens to the eczematous child when she develops a viral infection such as a cold or flu?

In my experience a viral infection will generally tend to aggravate the rash in a child with atopic dermatitis. However, on rare occasions I have also seen patients who for some inexplicable reason have *fewer* skin symptoms and complaints at this time.

What role do emotions play in the life of a child with atopic dermatitis?

Any time you are dealing with a chronic medical condition such as atopic dermatitis, the emotions must invariably be considered. Frustration, anxiety and anger all tend to aggravate the child's condition and make the rash significantly worse. For some children it may even be necessary to consider a mild tranquillizer. I have rarely had to prescribe such drugs. Sometimes I recommend that the parent take the tranquillizer so that he or she can cope with the severely eczematous child. Certainly a calm, stable atmosphere in the home is a worthy goal to aim for that will exert a definite and undeniably therapeutic effect on most children.

CHAPTER TWELVE

Allergies of the Ear and Eye

ALLERGIC CONDITIONS OF THE EAR

A three-year-old named Lesley was recently brought to my consulting room for an allergy evaluation. Lesley's chief problems, her parents explained to me, were her inability to get along with her nursery school classmates and poor language development. In reviewing Lesley's medical history I found that she had been suffering with recurring ear infections that required frequent antibiotic treatment. After repeated episodes of this condition, Lesley's doctor began to suspect that there might be an underlying allergic problem, so she was referred to me.

Lesley's physical examination revealed that there was fluid trapped behind her eardrum in the middle ear. A subsequent hearing test gave evidence of a low-grade hearing loss in both ears. Lesley, it seemed, had a condition known as serous otitis, or more technically, otitis media with effusion (OME). The decrease of hearing that resulted from the fluid accumulation was clearly interfering with both her language development and her ability to relate to her classmates.

In an attempt to get rid of the accumulated fluid a variety of antihistamines and decongestants were prescribed. Unfortunately, Lesley had only a partial response to the medicines and finally had to have the fluid drained from the middle ear by a procedure known as a myringotomy. A tiny incision is made in the eardrum (tympanic membrane) and the usually thickened fluid is removed by a suction machine. Drainage tubes (tympanostomy tubes, also known as grommets) are then left in place to make sure that the fluid doesn't reaccumulate. These tubes can remain and function well for twelve to eighteen months; they can then be easily removed by an ear, nose and throat specialist. In Lesley's case, within two weeks, according to her parents and her nursery school teacher, she was 'an entirely new child'. All symptoms, both physical and psychological, had disappeared.

This made us all proud, of course, but nothing had really been wrong with the bright child's developmental and emotional skills from the start. She had been suffering from a low-grade hearing loss, and because of this her inability to communicate with the outside world made her angry, frustrated and handicapped.

Lesley's story illustrates an important point: a physical problem can have a significant social and psychological impact on a person's life. Parents and doctors should consider possible unrecognized problems involving the eyes and ears in the case of any child not progressing normally at home and in school. The insidious thing about such conditions is that parents are not usually trained to recognize their symptoms and, of course, the child is too young to verbalize them and may be unaware of them, too. In this chapter we will examine a number of ear and eye ailments, both to provide parents with criteria for identifying them and as an aid for both parent and child in dealing with them.

Before getting into the hows and whys of childhood hearing loss problems, let's take a look at the anatomy of the ear and get a quick overview of how it functions. The human ear is divided into external, middle and inner sections.

The external ear This is the shell-shaped part of the ear visible from the outside. It consists of the auricle, which collects air vibrations resulting from sounds in the environment and the auditory canal, which transmits these vibrations to the middle ear.

The middle ear, or tympanum This section is normally filled with air. It houses the eardrum (tympanic membrane) and is connected to the nasopharynx at the back of the throat by means of the eustachian tube. Within its depths, as can be seen in Figure 9, there is a chain of three small movable bones called the stapes, incus and malleus. When air vibrations strike the eardrum they set in motion these bones, which then transmit the vibrations to the inner ear.

The inner ear or labyrinth In this final portion of the ear a link-up is made with the auditory nerve. This nerve then transmits these vibrations directly to the brain, where they are decoded and interpreted as specific sounds. The semicircular canals are involved in the equilibrium or balance mechanism of the body. The cochlea is a resonating chamber helping us to distinguish differences in sounds.

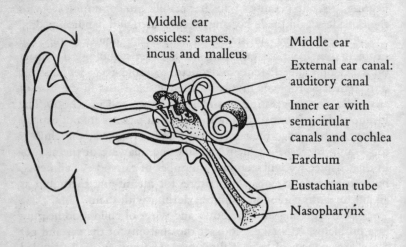

Middle ear ossicles: stapes, incus and malleus

Middle ear

External ear canal: auditory canal

Inner ear with semicirular canals and cochlea

Eardrum

Eustachian tube

Nasopharynx

Figure 9   Cross-section of a normal ear

ALLERGIC AND NONALLERGIC EAR PROBLEMS: TELLING THEM APART

Usually the ear is a highly sensitive and receptive organ, and we take its functions for granted. Trouble begins when the mechanism is thrown out of balance by disease or by an allergic reaction. The most common of such problems is acute otitis media or, as it is known to parents far and wide, the dreaded earache. This condition is *not* allergic, and parents should note the differences between its symptoms and those of genuine allergic conditions.

Acute otitis media (AOM) Just about all of us, young and old, have suffered from the pain of this common infection; in fact it is estimated that by the age of three, 70 per cent of all children have suffered from AOM at least once. The highest incidence takes place between the ages of six and twenty-four months. Allergy is not the cause of this infectious condition, and a positive family or personal history of allergy will not increase your child's risk of developing otitis media.

The most common symptoms of acute otitis media are the sudden onset of severe ear pain, usually associated with a fever. Occasionally a child suffering from this ailment will have neither of these signs, but such instances are an exception. Sometimes the ear feels hot to the touch and the child is irritable and out of sorts. Occasionally the pain becomes so strong that the patient cries and is inconsolable.

Otitis media is classified as acute if the symptoms clear up within three weeks, chronic if it lasts twelve weeks or more. Fluid accumulation in the middle ear – more on this below – may be associated with acute otitis media, though it is far more likely to occur when the condition is chronic.

Treatment with an appropriate antibiotic over a ten-to-fourteen-day period will usually cure the problem. A small number of children do develop accumulation of fluid behind the eardrum during the healing phase of AOM. This accumulation of fluid in the middle ear is known as an effusion.

If the effusion remains for several weeks, it becomes concentrated and eventually takes on a gluelike consistency. When this occurs, there will almost certainly be some degree of hearing loss. If an effusion persists, it may be necessary to make a small incision (myringotomy) in the eardrum and drain the thickened fluid from the middle ear. Quite often drainage (tympanostomy) tubes will be left in the eardrum to prevent fluids from reaccumulating. For this procedure an overnight admission to hospital may be necessary.

Parents should be on the lookout for any of the following situations that may indicate possible hearing loss due to an effusion in a child recovering from otitis media:

> The child continually increases the volume of the radio or record-player.

> The child seems unable to hear people who are speaking at a normal conversational level.

> The child's school work suddenly takes a dramatic turn
> for the worse.

If any of these situations are present, have your child's hearing
checked. Most doctors are equipped to do screening hearing tests
in their surgeries.

Secretory otitis media, or serous otitis Unlike acute otitis media,
serous otitis is sometimes linked to allergies and is prevalent in
children who suffer from allergic rhinitis. The persistence of fluid
in the middle ear may lead to hearing problems and must be treated
aggressively. While there are no accurate statistics to indicate what
percentage of children who develop serous otitis are actually
allergic, an educated guess based on information published in
medical journals tells us that approximately one-third have an
underlying allergic predisposition.

What causes serous otitis? We know that a significant increase
in the size of the adenoids can interfere with the normal drainage
functions of the eustachian tubes, thus leading to fluid accumulation in the middle ear. The mechanism by which an allergic
reaction in the nose leads to such middle-ear effusion works
roughly as follows: swelling of the nasal mucous membranes
extends into the region where the eustachian tube opens into the
nasopharynx (see Figure 9). The mouth of the eustachian tube may
become partially or completely blocked, depending on the amount
of allergic swelling in the area. This obstruction interferes with the
normal drainage of ear fluid, which then becomes trapped in the
middle-ear cavity. When allergic symptoms are treated with antihistamines or decongestants, the swelling in the nose decreases and
normal function of the eustachian tubes may be restored.

Symptoms of serous otitis revolve around hearing impairment, and, significantly, the fever and malaise found in AOM is
not present. Since the effusion in serous otitis is usually nonirritating, large amounts of the fluid can sometimes accumulate
without producing obvious symptoms. Common complaints
consist of statements such as 'My ears are blocked up', or 'It sounds
as if I'm hearing underwater', or 'It feels like my ears are dripping'.
Rarely is pain associated with serous otitis unless an infection
happens to be present as well.

When a child with this condition is brought to a doctor's surgery and examined, the doctor will most likely see 'bubbles' or even an actual fluid level behind the eardrum. Occasionally the fluid will exert so much pressure that the child's eardrum bulges outwards. Conservative treatment normally consists of decongestants or antihistamines, though I must tell you that several recent studies have questioned the effectiveness of these preparations, and prolonged accumulation of fluid usually requires either a simple drainage procedure (myringotomy) or the placement of drainage (tympanostomy) tubes in the ears.

Eustachian tube dysfunction When the eustachian tube, which connects the inner ear to the nasopharynx, doesn't function properly, one result is the accumulation of fluid in the middle ear.

The normal functions of the eustachian tube are:

to equalize the pressure between the nose, throat (nasopharynx) and middle ear

to block nasopharyngeal secretions from reaching the middle ear

to ventilate and supply oxygen to the middle ear

to serve as the pathway for the fluid normally produced in the middle ear to drain into the throat

If the eustachian tube fails to function properly because of either a physical obstruction such as a tumour (very rare) or what is termed abnormal potency, whereby the opening (ostium) of the eustachian tube (in the nasopharynx) either fails to close properly or opens at inappropriate times, there is a possibility of developing an infection or the accumulation of fluid in the middle ear.

Specific conditions that can lead to eustachian tube dysfunction include the following:

unrepaired cleft palates in infants

submucous cleft palates

divided uvula (the fleshy mass of tissue suspended from the centre of the soft palate over the back of the tongue) tumours involving the middle ear

certain degenerative muscle disorders

SPOTTING HEARING PROBLEMS EARLY

Now to the heart of the matter: how to recognize the symptoms of a low-grade hearing loss. What should you as a parent be on the lookout for in order to minimize the possibilities of this hazard?

During the first year of life a child who is unreasonably irritable, who sleeps poorly and who doesn't react appropriately to loud noises may be suffering from hearing impairment.

During the first two to three years, a delay in the development of normal speech patterns may be indicative of hearing difficulties.

In older children any of the following behaviour patterns can be tip-offs to low-grade hearing difficulties:

slow language development

the need to have statements repeated several times

lack of attention and concentration

frequent disobedience

complaints of popping noises in the ear, dull earaches, or a sensation of fullness in the head

a tendency to turn the volume of the radio or TV up inordinately loud

a tendency to speak too loudly

an inability to hear the phone ring or to hear the voice on the other end when picking it up

disobedience, disinterest and boredom in school; under-achievement in general

If several of these symptoms are present simultaneously, it should alert parents to the possibility that something more than childish laziness or contrariness is at the heart of the matter. If you have suspicions, don't hesitate to bring your child to the doctor's surgery for a hearing evaluation.

To avoid the development of middle-ear problems, never place infants in postures or positions that make it possible for them to aspirate fluid into the eustachian tube. Propping a bottle or using a poorly ventilated bottle teat are two situations that may lead to aspiration of fluid into the eustachian tube.

UNDERGOING A HEARING EVALUATION TEST

What procedures await your child when brought to the doctor's surgery for a hearing evaluation? First, as always, the doctor will review your child's personal and medical history. Then a physical examination will follow, focusing on the ears.

The doctor will examine your child's ears with a piece of equipment called a pneumatic otoscope. This is the standard otoscope to which a tube fitted with a rubber air bulb is attached. Squeezing the bulb when the otoscope is placed in the ear forces air against the tympanic membrane. This will cause the eardrum to move, and the doctor can tell if there is fluid behind the drum by the way it moves in response to the change in air pressure. The examination is called pneumatic otoscopy. The doctor may also place a vibrating tuning fork near the ear to check for hearing loss. A somewhat more sensitive method, designed to see how accurately the eardrum receives sound vibrations, is tympanometry. It is administered by means of a small apparatus called the tympanometer. The test is quick, painless and is especially valuable for evaluating the hearing of children six months or older. Of all the hearing tests given at the doctor's surgery, the most accurate is called audiometry. This procedure is generally administered to children over five years old. It is carried out in a quiet room where the child is asked to indicate when he hears sounds of different wavelengths piped into his ears. The response to these sounds is then analysed and evaluated, the result providing a highly accurate profile of the patient's ability to hear at a variety of sound levels. Occasionally an X-ray of a child's neck will be performed in order to check the size of the adenoids. If the adenoids become enlarged they may produce obstruction at the mouth of the eustachian tube, causing fluid to accumulate in the middle ear.

When fluid build-up in the middle ear is unresponsive to medical treatment, it will be necessary to remove the trapped secretions from behind the tympanic membrane. This is done by making a tiny incision in the eardrum, a procedure known as a myringotomy. The thickened secretions are then sucked out with a syringe; this relieves the pressure on the middle ear and provides a specimen that can be sent for appropriate bacteriological study. Occasionally this procedure will be performed in a doctor's consulting room, though more commonly it is done in a hospital.

TREATMENT FOR SEROUS OTITIS

Once the diagnosis of serous otitis has been made, environmental measures for the control of allergy such as those outlined throughout the book should be used for a child suffering from allergic ear problems. It is especially important to maintain adequate humidity in the child's immediate environment.

Now for specific treatment plans:

Antibiotics If any evidence of bacterial infection appears either as general symptoms (fever, malaise) or during a physical and laboratory examination (a red, painful eardrum, a positive bacterial culture) a ten-to-fourteen-day course of treatment with any appropriate antibiotic will be required.

Antihistamines/decongestants There is no consensus among allergists on how effective these medications really are in relieving serous otitis. My own experience indicates that an antihistamine, a decongestant or a combination preparation can *in some cases* provide symptomatic relief. A wide variety of these drugs is available over the counter at any chemist's. However, before starting your child on *any* course of treatment, please consult a doctor.

Topical decongestants and steroids A word of caution here: the prolonged daily use of nonprescription nose drops and sprays such as Afrazine, Antihistine, Privine, Otrivine and Neophryn (to name only a few) will *worsen*, not improve, both nasal and middle-ear symptoms. Such medications should be used for no longer than three to five days at a time and then discontinued (for a more thorough discussion of this matter, see page 157). Cortisone nasal sprays (Syntaris, Beconase, Rhinocort) are quite effective in reducing both swelling and inflammation in the nasal passageways. These preparations are poorly absorbed, highly surface-active forms of cortisone. This means that they work where they are sprayed (in the nose) and are rarely absorbed into the body. The likelihood that they will cause the types of undesirable side effects associated with prolonged oral use of cortisone is very, very small. Of course they should be used only as recommended by your doctor and only for as long as necessary.

Surgery If the various medical treatments outlined so far fail to clear up middle-ear problems caused by serous otitis, it may be necessary to consider surgical treatment.

Most common among such operations is the insertion of a small curved plastic or Teflon tube through the eardrum, the purpose being to drain secretions from behind the middle ear and to equalize the pressure on both sides of the eardrum. This surgical procedure, though somewhat simple, may require an overnight stay in hospital. The tube implanted in the ear during the operation may remain in place for weeks, and more usually months, until all infection has disappeared and hearing is restored. The operation is known as a myringotomy with placement of tympanostomy tubes.

A second surgical procedure that may also be recommended is an adenoidectomy. If a child's adenoids become so enlarged that they cause compression of the mouth of the eustachian tube (with obstruction and a consequent build-up of fluids in the middle ear), then this operation is clearly indicated. One word of caution, however: there is no guarantee that the adenoids will not grow back after they have been removed.

Finally, it is very difficult for both the parent and the doctor to know exactly what course this condition will take in any given child. Will it resolve itself over a period of weeks and months without any treatment? Perhaps, but not always. What effect will a partial hearing loss have on the child's development years? We do not know. No doubt it will have *some* negative effect, but just how great will this be?

While none of these intangibles can be precisely measured, it is my feeling that during the childhood years *any evidence whatsoever* of hearing loss, no matter how slight, should be given immediate and vigorous treatment to insure against a potentially permanent handicap. Whenever the health of a primary sense organ is involved, none of us can ever afford to take a wait-and-see attitude.

ALLERGIC CONDITIONS OF THE EYES

Alicia, aged six, becomes impossible to live with from late spring to late summer. Every morning she awakens with red, swollen eyes and angry temperament to match. She constantly complains that her eyes are itching, and whenever she goes outdoors her eyes swell up. There is simply no relief from this burdensome routine until late autumn.

Roger, an eleven-year-old, has had severe allergy symptoms during the spring and summer for several years. He regularly complains of an uncontrollable itching sensation around his eyes and the feeling that there are pebbles under his eyelids. He has become so sensitive to sunlight that whenever he goes outside he must wear dark glasses.

Cynthia, aged thirteen, has suffered from severe atopic dermatitis since she was four. Over the past several months she has complained that the quality of her vision is becoming impaired. An examination at the ophthalmologist's consulting room revealed early evidence of cataract formation.

Do you recognize any of these symptoms in your own child? Each has eye discomfort caused by allergic conditions. Alicia suffers from allergic conjunctivitis caused by sensitivity. Roger is a victim of vernal conjunctivitis. Cynthia's cataracts are a very unusual complication that can occur with severe atopic dermatitis. Of the three conditions, allergic conjunctivitis is the most prevalent, followed at a good distance by vernal conjunctivitis. Fortunately, cataracts resulting from atopic dermatitis are relatively rare.

Allergic conjunctivitis This allergic eye-disease is usually associated with allergic rhinitis. It may occur as an acute explosive reaction that involves either one or both eyes and can become a chronic problem.

The acute form produces sudden swelling of the conjunctiva (white portion of the eye) along with redness and profuse weeping. Frequently these children have an exquisite sensitivity to light (photophobia) and are extremely uncomfortable. They certainly require immediate medical attention.

The chronic form of allergic conjunctivitis is less likely to cause reddened, weeping eyes and more likely to produce eyes that are itchy and dry with blurred vision and increased light sensitivity. The white portion (conjunctiva) of the eye may have a finely granular or roughened appearance (if your child will let you close enough to take a look). Treatment for atopic conjunctivitis consists of both local and systemic medications. A combination of a vaso-constrictor and antihistamine, xylometazoline and antazoline sulphate (Otrivine, Antistin) is highly effective in controlling both the acute and chronic forms and is frequently prescribed. Steroid-based ointments and drops are also effective for serious cases. Cortisone preparations may be of great benefit to patients suffering from eye ailments, but if they are used for long periods of time without careful medical supervision, *severe ophthalmic complications can result*. It is my feeling that an ophthalmologist should be involved *whenever* cortisone eye preparations are prescribed and that the patient should be *closely monitored* to ensure that unaccept-able side effects do not develop.

Oral antihistamines are commonly prescribed for allergic conjunctivitis (see page 158 for a discussion and Table 7 for a list of the most commonly used antihistamines). These drugs are readily available and have an excellent safety record in the treatment of this condition. Finally, the newest and perhaps most promising medication on the market is a cromoglycate solution of sodium (see page 58) called Opticrom. Like all forms of sodium cromo-glycate, this drug works as a prophylactic agent, meaning that it is effective only if administered *before* eye symptoms develop. Side effects are almost nonexistent when the drug is used correctly; therefore Opticrom can be taken for long periods of time.

Vernal conjunctivitis This disorder is a relatively uncommon form of conjunctivitis that plagues sufferers in the spring and summer months. The exact cause is unknown. Children with vernal conjunctivitis complain of a severe itching involving both eyes and of the feeling that something is somehow 'stuck' in their eyes. Frequently a doctor will diagnose this condition by inverting the child's upper eyelid and searching for a characteristic cobblestone appearance, which looks exactly as the word suggests: small, hard, stonelike bumps encrusted on the inner side of the upper eyelid. Blurred vision and extreme sensitivity to light complete this ailment's unpleasant list of symptoms. Many more males than females have this condition.

Even in extremely stubborn cases, vernal conjunctivitis fortunately tends to clear up by itself before a child becomes an adult. Topical steroids are the most effective medications for treating this frustrating condition, but their use must be *scrupulously monitored* by an eye specialist. Most other ophthalmic medications are simply not very effective in this situation and at best will produce temporary symptomatic relief.

Conjunctivitis associated with atopic dermatitis The eyelids in this form of conjunctivitis may be thickened and very dry with a conspicuously 'cracked' appearance. Occasionally there will be wet, weeping lesions. The itching associated with this condition is severe and persistent compared with the conjunctivitis that accompanies hay fever. The cobblestone lesions, seen on the inner surface of the upper eyelid in vernal conjunctivitis, may show up on the lower lid in the atopic variety. In severe cases the cornea can become involved with the production of ulcers and cataracts; fortunately these are rare. (A complaint of severe light sensitivity should alert you to the possibility that corneal involvement may be taking place.) If such symptoms persist, consult a doctor *immediately*.

Treatment with the Opticrom and topical steroids generally proves effective in symptom control.

Contact dermatitis is a condition that not infrequently involves the eye. In this situation, the eyelids rather than the conjunctiva are primarily attacked. As discussed in the contact dermatitis section, there are many possible causes for the development of this itchy, scaling rash. Not uncommonly, teenage girls have this problem because of sensitivity to either eye make-up or nail polish.

Treatment consists of avoidance of the sensitizing substance and the use of mild strength steroid creams applied carefully to the eyelids. As always, before using any medicine, call and at least discuss the situation with the doctor.

QUESTIONS AND ANSWERS ABOUT EAR AND EYE ALLERGIES

Can permanent damage be done to the ear after a myringotomy?

A myringotomy consists of making a small incision in the tympanic membrane for the purpose of removing fluids trapped in the middle ear. The procedure is usually performed in a hospital, though it can also be done in a well-equipped otolaryngologist's (an ear, nose and throat specialist's) consulting room. The incision heals easily and completely, and there should be no subsequent problems of any kind. Certainly, under normal conditions there will be no permanent damage.

After a drainage tube (tympanostomy) has been removed from the ear, will the hole heal completely?

In most cases the incision in the tympanic membrane made to accommodate a drainage tube will close spontaneously. In a very small number of cases, usually those in which the patient has suffered severe repeated ear infections over a prolonged period of time, the damage done to the eardrum by these infections may cause the hole to remain permanently open. Even if this situation develops, it does not pose a particularly serious problem and it rarely interferes with a child's ability to hear.

If chronic serous otitis remains untreated, will this create the possibility of hearing loss?

If fluid is allowed to remain trapped in the middle ear for long periods of time, I believe the potential for hearing damage certainly exists. What happens is that the fluid becomes progressively thicker so that eventually the child ends up with a condition known rather graphically as 'glue ear'. In this case a degree of hearing loss almost always results. With the proper treatment in most cases – medical, surgical or both – the problem can be corrected.

What symptoms are most commonly associated with eye allergies?

Itching, weeping and redness of the eyes are the most characteristic. Dark circles under the eyes, the so-called allergic shiners, are also typical, for children with both nasal allergies and eye allergies. Whatever the case, always consult your doctor if eye symptoms of any kind persist. Certain infections cause symptoms similar to those produced by allergy, but their treatment is quite different.

Can a child's sight be permanently damaged if the eyes become swollen shut during an allergic reaction?

Although a youngster who is unable to open his eyes owing to an allergic reaction may become quite terrified, rest assured there will be no residual visual impairment once the external swelling has responded to appropriate treatment. Such treatment normally consists of oral antihistamines, decongestant/antihistamine eye drops, and cold compresses applied to the swollen eyes. Cortisone drops can be very effective for this type of reaction.

The white portion of my child's eyes has become so swollen that it actually bulges out of the eyes. How dangerous is this?

The white portion of the eye, the conjunctiva, can become dramatically swollen after exposure to almost any allergen – for example, pollen or contact with a household pet such as a dog or cat. If such swelling occurs, the allergist should be contacted immediately. Treatment with an oral antihistamine, topical steroids and local vasoconstrictor eye drops will normally control the situation. There is almost no chance that permanent eye damage can result from such a reaction.

CHAPTER THIRTEEN

Parents Beware: Controversial Practices in the Field of Allergic Medicine

One of the questions I am frequently asked by parents is how the different tests and procedures used by allergists are actually developed, tested and made safe. My answer is that the techniques commonly used in the diagnosis and treatment of allergic conditions are accepted by the medical profession *only* after they have been scientifically proved to be effective. This method, I tell them, is the heart and soul of all good science and is especially crucial to the development of all worthwhile advances in the field of medicine. Among its fundamental premises are the following concepts:

A procedure is valid only when its results can be consistently duplicated by individuals working independently of one another and all possibility that these results are due to coincidence, accident or placebo effect has been ruled out.

Final conclusions regarding the effectiveness of a specific diagnostic procedure or medical treatment programme can be reached only after analysing data from a large number of patients. This information must be statistically evaluated before recommendations are made to the medical profession and the general public.

With these guidelines as the foundation of medical experimentation, enough clinical and laboratory experience has been accumulated through the years to provide allergists with a variety of effective diagnostic techniques and therapeutic approaches for the management of allergic patients.

It would, of course, be immodest and incorrect for allergists to claim that their present methods for treating allergic diseases cannot be improved upon. They can, and they will. What is most important to understand is that new procedures will be accepted by the mainstream of medical practitioners *only* after they have been *proved* to be safe and effective.

In practical terms this means that a doctor in one part of the country using a certain procedure and one in another part, employing the same method will, under similar circumstances, obtain similar results. These doctors are in effect enjoying the benefits of the same principle, the principle of objective experimentation via the scientific method.

At the risk of sounding like a textbook writer for a moment, let's look a little more closely at this notion of the scientific method, because I want you to gain at least a passing awareness of how this important principle works. Why? So that if in the future you see a doctor who promises to clear up your child's allergic problem with a special diet or a new type of serum, you will be knowledgeable enough to ask the appropriate questions. If the doctor is unwilling to answer your questions, attempts to give you highly technical explanations or becomes evasive, you are probably with the wrong doctor!

Two main questions underlie the issue of medical legitimacy. How do medical research scientists determine that a laboratory procedure or new form of treatment is safe, reliable and effective? If we compare a traditional allergist and a doctor who uses what might be called controversial practices, what differences might we find in the manner in which they evaluate new treatment methods or testing procedures?

First, a description of the classical approach. Without becoming too technical, a step-by-step description follows of what a research scientist must do concerning the definition, observation, testing, evaluation and description of a new medical technique before this is accepted for general use by the medical community.

Hypothesis The hypothesis represents the concept or idea behind the procedure. This concept may involve a notion for the development of a laboratory test or for a new method of treatment. The hypothesis should be clearly stated and based as fully as possible on previously established knowledge and information.

Procedures and test materials The exact steps and materials necessary to perform the test must next be outlined very precisely. Such an outline will enable other technicians working anywhere in the world to duplicate the same test procedures.

Subjects If the test requires patient participation, a specific description of the study group should accompany all information concerning technique and chemical reagents. This permits other investigators to compare equal patient groups when evaluating the diagnostic or treatment procedure.

Test and control groups When it is time to perform clinical trials of the new procedure, two groups of subjects approximately the same in size, age, sex and degree of illness are chosen, the first for actual testing, the second as a so-called control group. For example, if we are testing a new asthma medicine, the test group will be given a pill that actually contains the new medicine. The second group, the control group, will receive pills that look exactly like the medicine but which actually contain none of the active ingredient. The reactions of both groups will be analysed and compared. Of course, neither group is told which is the control group.

Random selection When the entire population of test subjects has been assembled, the group will be divided into control and test sections by means of a statistical random selection procedure. In this way no claims can be made that subjects in one group were substantially different – more ill, more healthy, older, younger – from subjects in the other.

Evaluation When the study has been completed, the findings are collected and subjected to statistical analysis. In this way it becomes possible to determine if the results occurred by chance alone or were a consequence of the new item or technique being tested. This step is a critical one in analysing any new product or test method.

Results The final step is the publication in a medical journal of the entire study, including both the analysis and conclusion. Before this article can appear in print, it must first be passed through the final test: a written review by experts in the field. Once it has been put through these demanding paces, then and only then should it be released to the public.

THE FALLACY BEHIND THE ANECDOTE

As you can see, the demands made on medical researchers are rigorous and extremely objective; and well they should be, as the outcome of these tests involves significant matters of health and disease. Indeed, it can be said that any medical procedure that has not been put through this sequence of tests is unproven and should not be commercially available to the general public.

Unfortunately, there are a number of such unproven procedures and clinical practices in use today, several of which have recently achieved a degree of attention – if not respectability – within limited sectors of the medical community. The differences between these controversial practices and those which have become standard among allergists are significant and stem principally from the question of *proof*. What exactly does this mean? As I stated earlier, the scientific method requires that data obtained from group experiments be mathematically analysed by the latest in statistical methods before it can be certified for use on patients. This is in keeping with the scientific method. On the other hand, doctors who use what have been termed controversial procedures rely on quite another system of reporting which, in the opinion of most doctors, falls far short of objectivity. It is the so-called anecdotal method.

Anecdotal? In fact we have all heard such reports, stories about how at such-and-such a clinic doctors have had a 75 per cent recovery rate for cancer, about how Dr P—— has healed thousands of cases of incurable arthritis with his secret elixirs, and so forth. Technically, an example coming directly from a doctor might read as follows: 'In my experience, nine out of ten patients taking drug X have shown definite clinical improvement.' This sounds good, but where is the information regarding the use of a control group? Where is the statistical analysis? Where are the reviews and opinions by experts in the field? Where are the other doctors who have used the same methods and derived the same satisfactory results? Usually they are absent. All we have is one doctor's testimony, plus the testimony of a number of patients all or any of whom may have been cured by suggestion, by the body's natural healing processes, by accident, by the placebo effect, by half a dozen variables, none of which was actually brought about by the specific procedure itself.

The fact is that a single doctor's experience with a procedure can *never* stand alone as adequate medical testimony. The controversial procedure in question may indeed work, it may indeed cure; but then again, it may only *seem* to work. How can we tell the difference when a handful of practitioners have claimed wonderful results with the method while others simply cannot achieve the same success? If there is only anecdotal evidence in support of an otherwise unproven technique, a new patient should think it out very carefully before agreeing to undergo testing or treatment using an undocumented method. I believe, in fact, that more harm has been done to patients on both an emotional and financial level by the false raising of hopes than the possible small good such methods may have contributed through the placebo effect.

CONTROVERSIAL PRACTICES IN ALLERGIC MEDICINE

CYTOTOXIC TESTING

Cytotoxic testing is a procedure that requires the taking of approximately two teaspoonfuls of blood (10cc) from the patient. In the laboratory the white blood cells are separated from the red cells and the serum; a portion of the patient's white cell suspension is placed on a slide along with a specific dried food allergen – say, for peanut. A few drops of fluid are added and the slide is observed under a microscope. So far, so good. A positive reaction indicating a 'peanut allergy' can then supposedly be determined by what happens to the white blood cells. If they change their usual shape, slow down their normally active motion or disintegrate, an allergic sensitivity to that particular food is said to be proved.

It all sounds great – if only it were true. Today this test is being performed by laboratories and individual doctors in many of the major metropolitan centres around the country. It has been extensively advertised in both professional and lay publications and is frequently reported as being a 'state-of-the-art technique' for diagnosing a whole list of supposedly 'allergic' symptoms – which is even more ironical, as this particular method has been known and written about for approximately forty years.

Where, in my opinion and in the opinion of other allergists, does cytotoxic testing go wrong? Generally speaking, the test is used to diagnose food allergies and to identify the symptoms that reputedly accompany them. These symptoms include headache, skin rashes, nausea and other responses not necessarily character-istic of allergic reactions, such as heart palpitations and chronic insomnia. Champions of cytotoxic testing go so far as to claim that many apparently unrelated symptoms such as stress, depression and even backaches can all actually be the result of allergic reactions to food. They maintain that cytotoxic testing will determine which of these foods is really to blame.

All this would all be well and good, if it were true. From a number of well-controlled studies, the following contrary facts have clearly emerged:

> Results of cytotoxic testing done on the same patient on two separate days produced entirely different clinical results.

> Technicians working in different rooms studying the same cytotoxic test slides under the microscope were unable to agree on the results.

> Test results were unable to differentiate between foods which caused a clinical allergy in a patient as compared with foods which caused no problems when eaten by the same patient.

> In California, a specimen of blood obtained from a cow was sent to a laboratory for evaluation. The report from the laboratory stated that the patient was indeed allergic – to milk!

Finally, in an evaluation of all the existing studies made to date, the American Academy of Allergy and Immunology, an organization composed of recognized specialists in the field of allergic medicine, concluded that cytotoxic testing is 'unproven, unreliable and without scientific basis'. The US Food and Drug Administration in April 1985 stated that cytotoxic testing is 'unreliable as a diagnostic test'.

AUTOGENOUS URINE IMMUNIZATION

This technique involves the intramuscular injection of a patient's own urine after the urine has been sterilized and filtered under laboratory conditions. If such a bizarre procedure sounds suspect, it is. Fortunately, this method is rarely used today, and indeed it should never be used. Not only is there absolutely *no* evidence that urine injections are beneficial for allergic conditions (or for any other conditions, for that matter), but using such a technique can make the patient a candidate for a dangerous kidney disease called nephritis. For this reason the American Academy of Allergy and Immunology has issued a warning stating that autogenous urine immunization techniques are potentially dangerous to your health. If you were – or are – considering such a procedure for your child, my only word of advice on the subect is: don't!

RINKEL METHOD

Those allergists who use the Rinkel technique, which is supposed to determine the safe starting dose as well as the highest maintenance level for an immunotherapy ('allergy jab') treatment programme, have not proved their claims.

At first glance, this may sound like a technical argument for doctors only, and to some extent it is. But the question directly affects the patient as well. For any individual, the maintenance or top dose that the Rinkel method states is appropriate is far too weak to provide the patient with positive results. If your child is about to begin an immunotherapy programme, which usually takes years to complete, you as the parent need to know that the treatment will be effective. Indeed, the American Academy of Allergy and Immunology has analysed the results of several studies done on the Rinkel method and has come to the conclusion that the maximum dose suggested by this method is far too low to be medically useful. There was no evidence to prove that 'this method is an effective guide to determine the optimal therapeutic dose for immunotherapy.' It has even been found in at least one well-controlled study that there was no difference between a placebo and the ' "optimum therapeutic dose" called for by the Rinkel method'. This technique, under certain circumstances, recommends a top treatment dose that is so weak that the prospect of its helping the patient would be extremely unlikely.

PROVOCATION AND NEUTRALIZATION TESTING

As the name suggests, this method is designed to first provoke allergic symptoms in a patient (provocation) and then, in the second phase of treatment, to neutralize these symptoms and cause them to disappear entirely (neutralization). Those doctors who use this procedure claim that it is effective for both diagnosing and treating allergic conditions.

The first stage, the provocation part, is started either by the subcutaneous injection of the suspected allergen or by placing the extract directly under the child's tongue (sublingual). The allergen is administered in increasing strength until the supposed allergy-caused symptoms make their appearance.

Now for the neutralization stage. Here a 'neutralization dose' is given; this contains the same material used in the provocation dose, but in a much weaker dilution. This part of the procedure can be done either by placing the allergen under the tongue (sublingual neutralization) or by injecting the substance (subcutaneous neutralization). This extract may also be administered by injection or under the tongue and, according to its champions, it will quickly eliminate all allergic symptoms.

Once again, when this method was studied in a controlled fashion under appropriate laboratory conditions, investigators were unable to document its ability either to diagnose or to treat allergic conditions. By the way, this procedure has been recommended and marketed as a very effective way of diagnosing and treating food allergies. Unfortunately, it doesn't work! The

American Academy of Allergy and Immunology stated that provocation and neutralization methods are definitely 'unproven'. They also concluded that 'no known immunologic mechanism' could account for any symptoms being neutralized by the highly diluted antigen extracts used in this procedure. The Academy recommends that this test be considered an experimental procedure only and nothing more.

A FINAL WORD ON CONTROVERSIAL PRACTICES

I realize that it is extremely difficult for the parents of allergic children to read about so-called medical breakthroughs for asthma or so-called state-of-the-art food allergy therapies without being swayed. All I can advise is that before you spend your time, effort and money on one of these promised cures – and before you decide to opt for such methods at the expense of proven therapeutic procedures – you do a little investigating on your own.

The best person to ask is your own family GP. He should be able to tell you if it is a recognized medical procedure. If it is a very new procedure he may not be fully conversant with it, but he should be able to find out more than you will be able to on your own. He should know where to start asking. One of the difficulties is that some GPs are very conservative in their approach to 'fringe medicine' and are dismissive of anything new and outside their experience. However, the younger GPs are more open-minded and willing to look into the possibilities of acupuncture, homoeopathy and other unorthodox techniques.

CHAPTER FOURTEEN

Allergic Emergencies

One of the most frightening medical experiences for patient, parents and doctor is a generalized allergic response, technically known as an anaphylactic reaction. This is a true medical emergency, during which the patient develops intense generalized itching, swelling of virtually any part of the body – especially the face, tongue and throat – along with severe breathing problems. If untreated it can lead to shock, severe respiratory distress and death. Over the past twenty years I have treated children who were in anaphylactic shock; certain cases stand out clearly. One of them, a seven-year-old boy named Larry whom I had known for six months or so, was brought to my office twenty minutes after being stung by a yellow jacket (an aggressive stinging insect prevalent in the United States). Normally a bright penny of a boy, Larry now resembled a grotesque caricature of himself, his face swollen to practically twice its normal size, his skin covered with giant hives that itched uncontrollably, his lungs so congested that each breath had become a laboured gasp.

Larry responded dramatically to treatment with adrenaline, oxygen and antihistamines, and within two or three hours he was on his way home. He had to stay on medication for several days after the episode, and the psychological shock of this life-threatening experience left its mark not only on Larry but on his entire family.

The point is that an anaphylactic reaction is a highly traumatic experience for *everyone*, patient, parents and attending doctor alike. The message from Larry's case history which you must never forget is that *immediate medical attention must be given as soon as possible after generalized symptoms appear.*

This point cannot be emphasized too strongly. Anaphylaxis is a very serious condition, even a potentially fatal one, and it must be attended to rapidly or serious consequences will almost certainly occur. Unless you have proper medical training and have the appropriate drugs at home to treat an anaphylactic reaction, get your child to the nearest doctor or hospital *as soon as possible*. You are courting potential disaster if you attempt to manage this situation without medical assistance. In this chapter I will provide you with information on the causes, course and management of acute allergic reactions, focusing specifically on anaphylaxis. You can then use this information to recognize an allergic emergency quickly and act on it.

RECOGNIZING AN ALLERGIC MEDICAL EMERGENCY

How frequently do anaphylactic reactions occur? While completely accurate statistics are not available, it is possible to review those figures that have been published to get a general idea of how prevalent this problem is.

Fatal anaphylactic reaction will occur yearly to approximately four out of every ten million people. This means that statistically, with a population of roughly 56 million in Great Britain, somewhere in excess of twenty people per year will die of anaphylaxis. The actual number is almost certainly a good deal higher.

The number of nonfatal anaphylactic episodes in Great Britain ranges from 50 to 500 times higher than for fatal anaphylaxis. This means there may be as many as 10,000 cases a year of anaphylactic shock. Allergies to penicillin have been estimated at between 1 per cent and 10 per cent, according to which authority you consult. Anaphylactic reactions are said to occur in between one to five courses in every 10,000.

Although 400–500 deaths per year have been attributed to anaphylaxis to penicillin in the USA, only twenty-two deaths have been reported to the UK Committee on Safety of Medicines between 1964 and 1983.

Fatal reactions resulting from X-ray contrast media are estimated between one in 40,000 injections to one in 140,000, so a median figure would be around one in 100,000 injections.

From these few figures it is clear that anaphylaxis is a significant problem. Let me stress again, however, that while severe it can usually be controlled if prompt appropriate medical treatment is received. We may, in fact, assume that many of these reported fatalities occurred because of the victim's inability to gain medical help quickly or because he failed to recognize the seriousness of his symptoms until it was too late.

What determines whether a particular anaphylactic reaction will be serious or moderate? Two factors: the degree of sensitivity which the person has to the specific allergen, and the route by which the allergen enters the body. The first rule speaks for itself. The second, in practical terms, means that a child who is allergic to penicillin runs a much greater risk of reaction if the penicillin is injected rather than taken by mouth, and that a substance taken intravenously is more likely to produce a rapid and violent reaction than one received orally.

The areas most commonly involved during a generalized allergic reaction include the respiratory tract, the skin, the gastrointestinal tract and the cardiovascular system. The symptoms associated with each of these organ systems are as follows:

RESPIRATORY TRACT

Runny nose with profuse, clear, watery discharge.

A sensation of swelling in the throat, as though the throat were closing up.

A hoarse voice.

A tight feeling in the chest and a progressive inability to draw air into the lungs.

A tight cough associated with shortness of breath and wheezing.

If the reaction continues without appropriate treatment, respiratory arrest can occur.

THE SKIN

While skin symptoms tend to be generalized, they often begin at the injection site in the form of a red, itchy rash.

Hives. These may be small, individual lesions, or they may flow together to cover entire sections of the body. Distortion and swelling of the facial features due to angioedema.

Severe generalized itching with a red rash over most of the body.

GASTROINTESTINAL TRACT

Severe abdominal pain and cramping caused by swelling in the intestinal tract.

Nausea.

Vomiting.

Explosive diarrhoea (which is sometimes bloody).

CARDIOVASCULAR SYSTEMS

A sudden drop in blood pressure.

Irregular heartbeat.

Cardiac arrest (during the most severe episodes).

OTHER SYMPTOMS

An indefinable sense of impending disaster, a strange feeling that something terrible is about to take place. This sensation may come over the patient even if the symptoms are not yet apparent.

Convulsions.

Death due to anaphylaxis in children is relatively rare; most fatalities of this kind take place among the adult population. When death does occur to youngsters, it is usually due to severe swelling of the throat (laryngeal oedema), which makes it impossible to breathe. It should be mentioned, too, that a patient can have a milder, nonfatal form of anaphylactic reaction. In fact, when generalized reactions do take place you can rest assured that if proper steps are taken, the vast majority of cases will be controlled without serious consequences.

Finally, a note on the difference between anaphylaxis and anaphylactoid reactions. Briefly, while the symptoms of an anaphylactoid reaction and those of an anaphylactic reaction are practically the same, the causes are different. Anaphylactoid reactions are not IgE antibody-mediated responses – that is, they do not involve an antigen–antibody reaction. From a clinical point of view there is no way to tell the difference between these two reactions. Treatment is the same for both situations, and the response to medication is similar.

HOW TO DEAL WITH AN ALLERGIC EMERGENCY

Two important questions about allergic emergencies:

> What can I do if I suspect that a family member is having an anaphylactic reaction?

> What should the doctor do for a person having an anaphylactic reaction?

First question first. As a parent, probably the best thing you can do for your child, besides learning to recognize symptoms in advance, is *not to panic*. There is nothing more frightening for a youngster than the awareness that his parents are uncertain how to respond to his problem. If *you* can't help me, she thinks to herself, who can? Thus, even if you are not entirely sure of how to handle this difficult situation, *act as if you are*, at least until medical help has arrived. Most of all, stay clear-headed, deliberate and sympathetic. Even if you are not calm, try to act that way. Your calmness will help your child.

As soon as you suspect that your child is having an anaphylactic reaction, here's what you must do:

> Give an antihistamine. Chances are there will be one somewhere in the medicine cabinet, especially if your child has a history of allergy.

> Observe your child for any swallowing difficulties (swelling of the throat or a change in voice quality) or problems in breathing such as shortness of breath or wheezing.

> If there is any evidence of respiratory distress or swallowing difficulty, get your child to a doctor's surgery or a casualty department, and do it *immediately*. This situation is dangerous – this is a true medical emergency!

> If there are no breathing or swallowing problems, and if a trip to a hospital is not required, stay in touch with your doctor for additional directions.

What if your child's symptoms become so severe that you must go to a hospital? What can you expect once you arrive? More or less the following:

> A doctor will quickly examine and evaluate your child to determine the severity of the symptoms.

> Treatment will be started. In most cases the drug adrenaline will be used first. The dose will be determined by the patient's weight.

> A second injection of adrenaline will usually be administered within twenty to thirty minutes after the first. (A

patient can be given up to three injections of adrenaline at twenty-to-thirty-minute intervals.) An antihistamine may also be given orally or by injection.

Most patients will respond dramatically to the adrenaline. If there is any evidence of cyanosis caused by insufficient oxygen reaching the bloodstream, oxygen may also be administered. This will be given either by a face mask or by nasal prongs fitted directly into the nose.

For the majority of patients, combined treatment with adrenaline, antihistamines and oxygen will bring the anaphylactic reaction under control. Patients will continue to take antihistamines until all symptoms have disappeared; this is usually for one to three days.

If outpatient treatment is not successful in controlling the symptoms, your child may have to be admitted to hospital for more intensive therapy. Such treatment usually entails the administration of intravenous medications to raise blood pressure and control wheezing. Cortisone preparations will also be given to decrease both the severity and the duration of symptoms. If a period of hospitalization is necessary, it will rarely exceed two or three days. Most commonly an overnight admission is sufficient.

WHAT CAUSES ANAPHYLAXIS?

Throughout this book I have referred to the types of generalized reaction which may result from various allergic conditions. For specifics on the causes and aetiology of these difficulties, I refer you to the various chapters on asthma, food allergy, skin conditions, rhinitis, insect stings and so on. To review the subject briefly the following list of biological and chemical substances, though certainly not all-inclusive, represents a majority of the major offenders:

insect venom (see Chapter Eight)

penicillin (see Chapter Ten)

allergy extract treatment materials (see Chapter Ten)

vaccines made from horse serum (see Chapter Ten)

X-ray contrast media (see Chapter Ten)

local anaesthetics of the ester type (see Chapter Ten)

foods such as milk, eggs, shellfish, nuts, chocolate and fish (see Chapter Nine)

aspirin (see Chapter Ten)

chemicals added to foods such as dyes, colourings, stabilizers, emulsifiers and preservatives (see Chapters Ten and Nine)

For an allergic individual, any of these substances can become the trigger for an anaphylactic reaction. Once someone in your family has had such a response, it is strongly recommended that he wear a tag or necklace identifying the allergy; information about Medic Alert bracelets can be found at most chemists'. Finally – and repeating what has already been said several times – in the event of an anaphylactic reaction, the most important things you or anyone else can do for the victim are the following:

stay calm

give an antihistamine

call the doctor

if the symptoms become progressively worse, take the patient immediately to the nearest hospital

This is the key to success in treating any allergic emergency – quick recognition followed by rapid response and prompt medical attention.

Appendix

A BREATHING EXERCISE FOR CHILDREN WITH ASTHMA

BELLY BREATHING

Children should do the belly-breathing exercise (Figure 10) sitting down. Stand behind your child and put your hands on his shoulders.

MASSAGE

Gently massage your child's shoulders, chest, and back. Rub gently in circular motions for several minutes until the child expresses relief or visibly relaxes. The purpose of massage is to have parents and children work together to help each other relax.

PRODUCTIVE COUGH

Give your child a tissue. Then ask her to take a deep breath to open the lungs and airways. Second, make her cough strongly to bring up mucus from deep inside her lungs. Third, remove the mucus with a tissue.

This works well early when wheezing isn't severe. Don't do coughing in the middle of a serious attack: do it early. The child can even do this at school if she finds a private place. Encourage your child and make sure she takes a deep breath, then a big cough. Encourage your child to cough up mucus, not just saliva.

Parents and children can work together to manage an attack at home by doing belly breathing, massage, and productive cough. Belly breathing can help the child relax during an asthma attack or as she takes a breather during exercise. Massage can be used as an alternative form of relaxation if the belly breathing is not working well for the child. The massage can be done in association with productive cough. The sequence of these relaxation exercises is dependent on the personal preference of the child, based on past experience.

Sit up straight in a chair.

Place both hands on your belly.

Breathe in slowly through your nose. As you take the air in, feel your belly blow up like a balloon. Keep your chest still.

Blow the air slowly out of your mouth through puckered lips. Feel your belly get small.

Repeat this exercise slowly ten times or until you get your breath back.

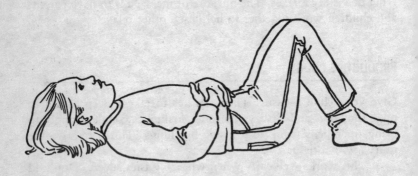

Figure 10 Belly-breathing exercise

SOURCE: C. H. Feldman and N. M. Clark, *Open Airways/Respiro Abierto: Asthma Self-Management Program*. National Heart, Lung, and Blood Institute, NIH Publication No. 84–2365.
SOURCE: National Heart, Lung & Blood Institute

FOOD FAMILIES

An allergy to one member of a specific food family may mean sensitivity exists to the other foods in the family. Certain families are more likely to have this characteristic, such as the pea and citrus families.

Food	Other food family members
Apple	Apple, pear, quince
Aster	Artichoke, chicory, dandelion, endive, lettuce, sunflower seeds, tarragon
Banana	Banana, plantain
Beet	Beet, spinach
Beech	Beechnut, chestnut
Buckwheat	Buckwheat, rhubarb, sorrel
Cashew	Cashew nuts, mango, pistachio nuts
Chocolate	Chocolate, cocoa, cola
Citrus	Citron, grapefruit, kumquat, lemon, lime, tangerine
Ginger	Cardamom, ginger, turmeric
Goosefoot	Beet, beet sugar, spinach, Swiss chard (*see* Beet)
Grains	Barley, cane, corn, millet, oats, rice, rye, sorghum, wheat, wild rice
Laurel	Avocado, bay leaves, cinnamon, sassafras
Lily	Asparagus, chives, garlic, leeks, onion, sarsaparilla
Mallow	Okra
Melon (Gourd)	All kinds of melon including watermelon, courgette, cucumber, marrow, pumpkin
Mint	Basil, mint, peppermint, rosemary, sage, spearmint
Morning glory	Sweet potato, yam
Mulberry	Bilberry, currants, gooseberry, mulberry

Mustard	Broccoli, Brussels sprouts, cabbage, cauliflower, horseradish, kale, mustard, radish, swede, turnip, watercress
Myrtle	Allspice, guava
Palm	Coconut, date
Parsley	Aniseed, caraway seed, carrot, celery, celery seed, coriander, cumin, dill, fennel, parsley, parsnip
Pea (Legume or Clover)	Acacia, black-eyed peas, licorice, lima beans, peanuts, peas, pinto beans, string beans, tragacanth
Plum	Almond, apricot, cherry, nectarine, peach, plum
Potato	Aubergine, bell peppers, cayenne peppers, chili peppers, paprika, potato, tomato
Rose	Blackberry, boysenberry, loganberry, raspberry, strawberry
Walnut	Butternut, hickory nut, pecan, walnut
Bird	Chicken, duck, goose, pheasant, guinea fowl, pigeon, quail, turkey; the eggs of these birds
Crustaceans	Crabs, crayfish, lobster, prawns, shrimps, squid
Fish	(Includes both fresh- and salt-water fish) Bass, catfish, flounder, halibut, perch, pike, salmon, sardine, trout, tuna, whitefish
Mammal	Cow, goat, horse, pig, sheep, and their meat, milk or by-products
Mollusc	Abalone, clam, mussel, oyster, scallops

FOOD ADDITIVES

AZO DYES USED AS FOOD COLOURING

E 102	Tartrazine
107	Yellow 2G
E 110	Sunset yellow FC (Orange Yellow S)
E 122	Carmoisine (Azorabine)
E 123	Amaranth
E 124	Ponceau 4R (Cochineal Red A)
128	Red 2G
E 151	Black PN (Brilliant black BN)
154	Brown FK
155	Brown HT (Chocolate brown HT)
E 180	Pigment rubine (Lithol rubine BK)

COAL TAR DYES (SYNTHETICALLY MADE DYES: AN OLD NAME)

E 104	Quinoline yellow
E 127	Erythosine BS
E 131	Patent blue V
E 132	Indigo carmine (Indigotine)
133	Brilliant blue FCF

ADDITIVES USED AS PRESERVATIVES WHICH CAN CAUSE SYMPTOMS

E 210	Benzoid acid
E 211	Sodium benzoate
E 220	Sulphur dioxide
E 250	Sodium nitrite
E 251	Sodium nitrate
E 320	Butylated hydroxyanisole (BHA)
E 321	Butylated hydroxytoluene (BHT)

ADDITIVES WHICH CAN CAUSE SYMPTOMS IN ASTHMATICS OR ASPIRIN-SENSITIVE PEOPLE AND MIGHT BE UNSUITABLE FOR CHILDREN

E 212	Potassium benzoate
E 213	Calcium benzoate
E 214	Ethyl 4-hydroxybenzoate (ethyl para-hydroxybenzoate)
E 215	Ethyl 4-hydroxybenzoate, sodium salt (sodium ethyl para-hydroxybenzoate)
E 216	Propyl 4-hydroxybenzoate (propyl para-hydroxy-benzoate)
E 217	Propyl 4-hydroxybenzoate, sodium salt (sodium propyl para-hydroxybenzoate)
E 218	Methyl 4-hydroxybenzoate (methyl para-hydroxy-benzoate)
E 219	Methyl 4-hydroxybenzoate, sodium salt (sodium methyl para-hydroxybenzoate)
E 310	Propyl gallate
E 311	Octyl gallate
E 312	Dodecyl gallate
621	Sodium hydrogen L-glutamate (monosodium glutamate: MSG)
622	Potassium hydrogen L-glutamate (monopotassium glutamate)
623	Calcium dihydrogen di-L-glutamate (calcium glutamate)
627	Guanosine 5'–(disodium phosphate) (sodium phosphate)
631	Inosine 5'-(disodium phosphate) (sodium inosinate)
635	Sodium 5'-ribonucleotide

Sources of Salicylates

Drugs

Actron
Alka Seltzer
Anadin
Antoin
Askit
Aspergan
Aspar
Aspellin
Aspirin
Aspro
Beechams Powders
Benoral
Caprin
Claradin
Codis
Cojene
Disprin
Doan's Backache Pills

Doloxene
Equagesic
Fennings
Genasprin
Hypon
Laboprin
Migravess
Mylogin
Nu-Seal Aspirin
Palaprin
Paynocit
Phensies
Powerin
Safapryn
Solprin
Trancoprin
Triadol
Veganin

Foods

Almonds
Apples
Apricots
Blackberries
Cherries
Currants
Gooseberries
Grapes

Nectarines
Oranges
Peaches
Pears
Plums
Quinces
Raspberries
Strawberries

BEVERAGES

Coffee

Cola drinks

Fruit juices

Tea, including Peppermint tea

Wine and most other alcoholic drinks

FLAVOURINGS

Oil of wintergreen

Spices and herbs, particularly aniseed, cayenne, celery seed, cinnamon, cumin, curry, dill, fenugreek, five-spice powder, garam masala, mace, mustard, oregano, paprika, rosemary, sage, tarragon, thyme, turmeric, vanilla

MISCELLANEOUS

Antiseptics

Chewing gum

Cosmetics

Lozenges

Mouthwash

Perfumes

Suntan lotion

Toothpaste

FOOD ALLERGY

Health food shops or special foods sections in your local supermarket are excellent sources for specialized food products. The organizations listed on page 320 will be able to help with information.

You can also find many diet and food books in your local library that will provide you with a more extensive and varied menu for dealing with your allergic child. Your local librarian can serve as an excellent resource for you.

In some instances you may have to seek the advice and guidance of a dietitian or nutritionist. Be certain that the person you choose has the proper credentials. A referral from your doctor is an excellent recommendation.

Of course your allergist will discuss any plans for dietary manipulation with you and make general recommendations regarding menu planning.

FOOD ALLERGY ELIMINATION DIETS

The choice of a specific elimination diet will depend on which food is suspected of causing the symptoms. As a general rule, a discussion with your doctor is recommended before making any major or prolonged diet changes. The elimination diets may be used to determine which food is a possible cause of symptoms. The most common sensitizing foods in order of frequency are egg, milk, seafood, nuts, seeds, chocolate, orange and tomato.

Two diets are listed. These contain entirely different foods with the exception of sugar, salt and gelatin. Common allergens are excluded with the exception of milk on Diet Two. The choice of diet depends on the history and skin tests. The diet you choose will depend on the foods you suspect. Choose the diet that has no foods which you suspect cause allergic symptoms in your child. If there is any food on the diet which you know disagrees with your child, omit it. The diet should be maintained rigidly for two weeks, unless symptoms are aggravated. If this occurs, or if there is no improvement, the other diet may be tried.

When improvement occurs, new foods are added at three-day intervals. Symptoms appearing on the addition of a food to the basic diet are the most significant evidence of food allergy. Such evidence should be checked by reintroducing the suspect food after at least a week's abstinence.

These diets are nutritionally inadequate and should not be maintained without change for longer than two weeks. Vitamins, minerals and drugs should not be taken without asking your doctor.

On Diet One, where milk is not allowed, meat should be given twice a day to ensure adequate protein. Calcium may be added. Foods containing preservatives should be avoided.

WHEAT-FREE DIET

Omit these foods.

Beverages

Malted milk, coffee substitutes, beer, ale.

Bread

All breads including rye, unless 100 per cent rye, oatmeal, nut breads, rolls, scones, biscuits, cakes, buns, crispbreads, wafers and crackers.

Table 14   Elimination diets

Diet One	Diet Two
Beverages	
Apricot juice	Apple juice
Lemonade	Grape juice
Pineapple juice	Prune juice
Tea	Coffee
	Milk
Cereal	
Pure corn	Rice
Meat	
Lamb, any cut	Beef, any cut
Pork, any cut	Chicken, any cut
(bacon, ham)	Veal, any cut
Vegetables	
Asparagus	Beets
Beans, all kinds	Carrots
Cabbage	Lettuce
Corn	Marrow
Sweet potato	Turnips

Table 14 Elimination diets–continued

Diet One		Diet Two
	Fruit	
Apricots		Apples
Banana		Grapes and raisins
Lemon		Plums
Pears		Prunes
Pineapple		
	Bread	
		100 per cent rye bread and wafers
	Fat	
Bacon fat		Butter
Mazola oil		Chicken fat
	Miscellaneous	
Apricot jam		Apple butter
Gelatin		Apple jelly
		Cider vinegar
Molasses		Cheese
Salt		Gelatin
Sugar		Grape jelly
		Salt
		Sugar

Cereals

All Bran	Ralston – regular, instant shredded
Bran Flakes	Shredded Wheat
Cocoa Pops	Shreddies
Crackles	Special K
Farina	Sugar Crisp
Fruit and Fibre	Sugar Smacks
Grapenuts	Total
Infant cereals	Weetabix
Nutrigrain	Wheat Flakes
Protein Plus	Wheat germ
Puffed Wheat	Wheaties
Raisin Bran	Whole Bran

Flours

Wheat flour in any form including granary, white or wholewheat.

Desserts

Cakes, biscuits, doughnuts, pies, ice cream cones, pastries, puddings and prepared mixes except those especially made without wheat.

Miscellaneous

Macaroni, spaghetti, noodles, vermicelli, and other pasta

Dumplings, griddle cakes, waffles, pancakes, French toast, pizza, ravioli

Commercial sweets that contain wheat

Gravies and sauces thickened with flour, commercial sauces made with wheat

Soups containing wheat or wheat products, including canned broth or consommé

Fish or meats prepared with flour, bread or biscuit crumbs, such as croquettes, meat loaf and stew thickened with flour

Commercially prepared meat, such as frankfurters, sausages and cold cuts where wheat may be used as a filler

Salad dressings – cooked or boiled – where flour is used for thickening.

Acceptable bread and other baked products can be made with all soy, rice, corn or potato flour or cornmeal; 100 per cent rye breads, crackers and wafers are available in some stores.

EGG-FREE DIET

Omit these foods.

Biscuits	custard, pumpkin, coconut, etc.
Breads prepared with egg	Custard
Cake	Doughnuts

Cake icing prepared with egg

Crackers prepared with egg

Cream-type pies, such as lemon,

Eggnog or other egg drinks

Fish or meat prepared with egg, such as meat loaf, croquettes, breaded meats

Foods containing albumin

French toast

Fritters

Griddle cakes

Hollandaise sauce

Ice cream

Macaroons

Marshmallows

Mayonnaise and salad dressings

Meringue

Eclairs

Eggs

Milk puddings containing eggs

Noodles

Pretzels

Ravioli

Soft sweets, such as chocolate cream, nougat or fondant

Soft rolls prepared with egg

Sweet rolls and pastries

Rusks

Tartare sauce

Vaccines made in egg, such as those used for influenza

Waffles

Yorkshire pudding

MILK-FREE DIET

Omit any foods and commercial mixes containing milk, dried milk solids, casein, lactalbumin or curds and/or whey.

Bread made with milk

Butter and margarine (unless kosher)

Cakes, sweets and biscuits made with milk or milk products

Caramels

Cereals prepared with milk

Cheese

Chocolates

Cocoa beverages

Crackers made with milk

Cream

Cream or soft pies

Cream sauce

Cream soup

Ice cream

Icing prepared with milk

Instant breakfast mixes

Instant cocoa mix

Malted milk

Milk

Milk, condensed

Milk, evaporated

Milk, powdered

Milk, skimmed

Milk puddings

Milk shakes

Ovaltine

Potato mashed with milk

Rusks

Creamed or scalloped foods	Sweet rolls and pastries
Custard	Vegetables with milk or
Doughnuts	cream
Gravies with milk and cream	Yogurt

This information is adapted from the Diet Manual of the Presbyterian Hospital in the City of New York at the Columbia-Presbyterian Medical Center.

ADDRESSES UK

SELF HELP AGENCIES

Action Against Allergy
43 The Downs,
London SW20 8HG   Tel. (01) 947 5082

Food & Chemical Allergy Association
c/o The Chairman,
Mrs Ellen Rathera,
27 Ferringham Lane,
Ferringham,
West Sussex B12 5NB   Tel. (0903) 41178

Medic Alert Foundation
11/13 Clifton Terrace,
London N4 3JP   Tel. (01) 263 8596

The Asthma Society
Friends of the Asthma Research Council,
300 Upper Street,
London N2 X4   Tel. (01) 226 2260

Invalid Children's Aid Nationwide
Allen Grahame House,
198 City Road,
London EC1V 2TH   Tel. (01) 608 2462

National Eczema Society
Tavistock House North,
Tavistock Square,
London WC1H 9SR   Tel. (01) 388 4097

National Society for Research into Allergy
PO Box 45,
Hinckley,
Leicestershire LE10 1JY

Food & Drink Federation
6 Catherine Street,
London WC2B 5JJ   Tel. (01) 836 2460

A booklet, *Look at the Label*, can be obtained from:

In England and Wales:

Ministry of Agriculture, Fisheries and Food
Publication Unit,
Lion House,
Willowburn Trading Estate,
Alnwick,
Northumberland NE66 2PF   Tel. 0665 602881

In Scotland:

Scottish Office
Foods Branch,
Room 40,
St Andrew's House,
Edinburgh EH2 3DE   Tel. 0315 540368

In Northern Ireland:

The Department of Health and Social Services
Medicines and Food Control Branch,
Annex A,
Dundonald House,
Upper Newtownards Road,
Belfast BT4 3SF   Tel. 0232 650111

Products

While listing these products and suppliers does not constitute an endorsement by the author or publisher, we hope that this guide will help you to find household and personal products that you and your child can use safely.

Air purifiers

Astec Ltd
31 Lynx Crescent,
Weston Industrial Estate,
Weston-Super-Mare,
Avon
BS24 9DJ   Tel. 0934 418685

Beta Plus
177 Haydons Road,
Wimbledon,
London SW19   Tel. (01) 543 1142

Coast Air
Unit 2,
Chilton Industrial Estate,
Mills Road,
Sudbury
Suffolk CO1D 6XX   Tel. 0787 76259

Patent Enterprises Ltd
PO Box 426,
Chipperfield,
Kings Langley,
Herts WD4 9PJ   Tel. 09277 60993

Bedding

Futon Co.
138 Notting Hill Gate,
W11 3QG   Tel. (01) 221 2032

Green Farm Nutrition Centre
Burwash Common,
East Sussex
TN19 7LX   Tel. 0435 882180

Keys of Clacton Ltd
Old Road,
Clacton,
Essex   Tel. 0255 424351

Cotton On
29 North Clifton Street,
Lytham,
Lancs
FY8 5HW   Tel. 0253 736611

Breathing aids – hay fever helmet and air cleaner (plastic bubble)

R. H. Hinchcliffe & Sons
39 High Street,
Pershore,
Worcs   Tel. 0386 555566

ADDRESSES AUSTRALIA

SELF-HELP AGENCIES

Allergy Association Australia

Allergy Association Australia is a self-help group for people suffering from allergies and sensitivities to substances in their environment whether ingested, inhaled or touched. AAA has helped to set up many branches whose various services include regular newsletters, discussion groups, dissemination of information, counselling on allergy problems. Guest speakers are invited to regular meetings. AAA also aim to co-operate with the medical profession and to support research into the causes and treatments of allergies.

Members of the Association have access to the bi-monthly newsletters and/or resources information. There are branches in all states. For more information, the main state associations are:

**Allergy Association Australia –
Victoria**
PO Box 298, Ringwood,
Vic 3134   Tel. (03) 720 3215

**Allergy Recognition and
Management Inc.
Allergy Association Australia –
Tasmania**
PO Box 604F, Hobart
Tas 7001   Tel. (002) 29 6047

Allergy Association – WA
c/o Ms Hilary Lane,
52 Dempster Street,
Karrinyup, WA 6018   Tel. (09) 447 5661

Allergy Association Australia – NSW
PO Box 74,
Sylvana Southgate,
NSW 2224

Allergy Association Australia – Brisbane North
PO Box 45,
Woody Point,
QLD 4019   Tel. (07) 283 4786

Allergy Association Australia – SA
37 Second Avenue,
Sefton Park,
SA 5083   Tel. (08) 269 3130

Allergies and Intolerant Reaction Association
PO Box 1780,
Canberra City,
ACT 2610

Sensitivity Awareness Organization
PO Box 66,
Kenthurst,
NSW 2154

Asthma Foundation of Australia

Asthma Foundation of New South Wales
1 Angel Place,
Sydney
NSW 2000   Tel. (02) 235 1202

Asthma Foundation of Victoria
2 Highfield Grove,
Kew
VIC 3101   Tel. (03) 861 5666

Asthma Foundation of Queensland
PO Box 394,
Fortitude Valley QLD 4006   Tel. (07) 527 677

Asthma Foundation of South Australia
Epworth Building,
33 Pirie Street,
Adelaide SA 5000   Tel. (08) 514272

Asthma Foundation of Tasmania
Hampden House,
82 Hampden Road,
Battery Point Tas 7000   Tel. (002) 237 725

Asthma Foundation of Western Australia
Suite 2,
Heytesbury House,
61 Heytesbury Road,
Subiaco WA 6008

Asthma Foundation of the Northern Territory
c/o PO Box 41326
Casuarina NA 5792

The above organizations run yearly camps for children between
the ages of eight and twelve who suffer from asthma. They also
have newsletters available to the public which deal with asthma
both in adults and children.

PRODUCTS

While listing these products and suppliers does not constitute an
endorsement by the author or publisher, we hope that this guide
will help you to find household and personal products that you
and your child can use safely.

Many products can be bought from chemists and health-food
stores. The following provide items directly or items not easily
available elsewhere.

Allersearch

Allersearch supply through pharmacies and direct to the public by mail order. They will provide mail lists and samples on request. Their range includes:

> Bedding for dust and mould allergies – duvet covers, mattress covers, pillow covers, etc.
>
> Sprays for containing dust, dust mites and mould
>
> Face masks – dust masks and charcostatic masks for chemical allergies
>
> Air cleaners – to eliminate pollen, dust, mould spores, pollutants, cigarette smoke, chemical fumes
>
> Allergo range of soaps, shampoo, laundry and dish-washing detergents for chemically sensitive people
>
> Ionizers
>
> Water purifiers
>
> Products for asthma sufferers – nebulizer pumps, peak flow meters.

Head Office:
Allersearch Asthma and Allergy Aids
8 Marco Avenue,
Revesby,
NSW 2212   Tel. (02) 771 6944

Agencies of Allersearch:
VIC: Allersearch, 82 Lewis St, Wantima, Vic 3152.
          Tel (03) 221 6011
QLD: Allersearch, Medical and Surgical Requisites, 50 Vulture St, West End, Qld 4101
          Tel. (07) 844 2966
WA: Allersearch, c/o Thomas Surgical, 12 Ellen Street, Subiaco, WA 6008
          Tel. (09) 381 5344

Allergy Aid Centre

Mail order service direct to the public. Catalogues supplied on request. Wide range of stock and will also search out items on request. Stock includes:

Bedding – sheets, pillowcases, duvet covers, blankets, mattress covers, etc.

Beds and mattresses

Face masks including activator charcoal masks

Herbonics range of soaps, laundry and dishwashing detergents for chemically sensitive people

Ionizers

Water purifiers and distilled water

Products for asthma sufferers – nebulizer pumps

Cosmetics – including Nutri-metic and Biochemical ranges

Foods

Furniture – made without glue, etc.

ADDRESSES NEW ZEALAND

Allergy Awareness Association Inc
PO Box 12–701
Penrose
Auckland

93 Waipapa Road
Hataitai
Wellington
203 Hoon Hay Road
Hoon Hay
Christchurch

Toxins Action Group
PO Box 35–453
Browns Bay
Auckland

Glossary

Words set in small capitals are defined elsewhere in the Glossary.

ADRENALINE A chemical produced by the human adrenal glands and frequently used to treat bronchial asthma and allergic emergencies.

AIR POLLUTION A major problem in most industrial and urban areas and an aggravating factor for those who suffer from respiratory allergies. Compounds such as sulphur dioxide and carbon monoxide are two of the many chemical substances that can precipitate asthma attacks in susceptible individuals.

ALLERGENIC Capable of causing an allergic reaction.

ALLERGENIC EXTRACT Substance employed in the diagnosis and treatment of allergic individuals. The most commonly used of these are water-based substances known as aqueous extracts. They are prepared by grinding and removing the fat from the original material, placing the allergenic portion of the material into an extraction fluid (most often a buffered salt-water solution), passing the material through a glass column (dialysing column), and sterilizing the final product; it is then ready for use as a diagnostic and therapeutic agent. A long-standing problem with allergenic extracts has been standardization: how to guarantee that one hundred units of company A's product – say, pollen extract – is equal to one hundred units of company B's product. This dilemma, as yet unresolved, can under certain conditions complicate the treatment of a patient who moves from one part of the country to another or who switches from one doctor to another.

A number of allergenic extracts will soon be commercially available which are chemically processed in such a way that fewer injections will be required in order for a patient to reach a maintenance dose. These injections will be given at less frequent intervals than those which come in aqueous extracts. They are called polymerized allergens.

Therapy by injections of allergenic extracts has virtually stopped in the UK because of the precautions recommended by the Committee on Safety of Medicines, but it is hoped that they will be able to start up again sometime in the future.

ALLERGEN Special type of ANTIGEN, i.e., any substance foreign to the human body, capable of triggering allergic symptoms in a sensitized person. Exposure to an allergen may come through contact with the skin, from ingestion, or from inhalation. Common allergens include mould spores, pollen grains from trees, grasses and weeds, dust, mites, danders, feathers, mouldspores and industrial and occupational dust substances. *See* ANTIGEN.

ALLERGIC IgE ANTIBODY An ANTIBODY that, when interacting with a specific ANTIGEN, is responsible for producing allergic reactions. For example, in order to develop symptoms of hay fever a person's body must first produce anti–grass IgE antibodies and then be exposed to the grass pollen. The reaction of these two substances will combine to cause the sneezing, streaming eyes and runny nose typical of hay fever. The human body is capable of producing multimillions of different antibodies; while most of us produce small amounts of IgE, allergic individuals have high levels in their bloodstream. The IgE level is a general indicator of a person's potential for developing allergic symptoms.

ALLERGIC BRONCHOPULMONARY ASPERGILLOSIS An unusual lung ailment which sometimes occurs in patients suffering from allergic asthma. The condition is caused by infection with a fungus called aspergillus.

ALLERGIC RHINITIS A complex of symptoms consisting of sneezing, runny nose, and itchy nose which may occur as a seasonal problem, called rose fever or hay fever, or as a year-round condition known as perennial allergic rhinitis.

ALLERGIC SHINERS Dark circles which form under the eyes, commonly seen in allergic children, caused by local swelling and a sluggish blood flow throughout the many capillary blood vessels surrounding the eyes.

ALLERGIST A doctor who usually has membership of the Royal College of Physicans and who has then specialized in allergy.

ALLERGOID An ALLERGENIC substance that has been chemically modified so that its ability to produce allergic reactions is significantly decreased, while its capacity to stimulate protective IgG antibody production remains unchanged. These materials are being studied today for possible use as immunizing agents for allergic patients.

ALLERGY A pathological reaction to environmental substances such as foods, pollens, dust and so on. The term was derived from the Greek words *allos* (other) and *ergon* (action). People who suffer from allergies develop an 'altered response' when exposed to specific environmental substances. This response is both protective (as an immune response) and harmful (it can cause a person to become hypersensitive). In common usage the term *allergy* has become synonymous with hypersensitivity.

ALVEOLI The small, balloonlike air sacs at the ends of the smallest air passageways in the lungs. Oxygen and carbon dioxide transfer takes place in the alveoli.

AMINOPHYLLINE A form of THEOPHYLLINE used in the treatment of bronchial asthma.

ANAPHYLACTOID A generalized reaction that mimics an anaphylactic response but is not caused by an allergic, IgE-mediated reaction. A common example is the response certain patients experience when injected with contrast media for X-ray studies, especially the media used for an intravenous pyelogram. See ANAPHYLAXIS

ANAPHYLAXIS A term used to define a severe, GENERALIZED ALLERGIC REACTION occurring either immediately or several hours after exposure to an ALLERGEN. Symptoms may include local or generalized hives or ANGIOEDEMA, persistent sneezing, continuous watery nasal discharge, shortness of breath, tightness in the chest, wheezing, swelling of the throat and larynx, a drop in blood pressure, unconsciousness and possibly death. These symptoms take place following the massive release of a variety of chemical substances, called MEDIATORS.

ANGIOEDEMA A localized swelling in the deeper layers of the skin generally caused by an allergic reaction. There is rarely any itching associated with angioedema. While typical areas of swelling include the lips, eyelids, feet and hands, angioedema can occur in virtually any part of the body. *See* URTICARIA

ANTIBODY A special type of protein manufactured by plasma cells in response to any foreign substance (or ANTIGEN) entering the body. Once produced, the antibody is capable of reacting only with its specific antigen. For example, in order to become sensitized to a cat, a dog or pollen, a child's body must first produce specific antibodies against cat, dog or pollen antigens.

Allergic antibodies are collectively found in a class of proteins called IgE. There are also other antibody types, a majority of them involved in the body's defence mechanism against infection. Most common of these is gammaglobulin or IgC. Other antibody groups are labelled IgA, IgM and IgD. *See* IMMUNOGLOBULIN

ANTIGEN Any foreign substance that causes specific antibodies to be produced in the body and has the capacity to stimulate an immune response. For example, exposure to dog antigen in a child may cause the production of antidog IgE antibodies in that child. During a lifetime the body is exposed to millions and millions of antigens. It responds by producing a specific antibody for each. *See* ANTIBODY

ANTIHISTAMINE A family of drugs used in the treatment of common allergic symptoms such as sneezing, runny nose, weeping eyes and itching. The many antihistamines on the market today come from five distinct chemical groups and a sixth group labelled miscellaneous. Antihistamines work by blocking the effect of the chemical substance histamine, which is manufactured and released by the body during an allergic reaction. *See* HISTAMINE

ANTISERUM An immunizing agent which contains antibodies and is used to prevent certain infections. For example, an antiserum prepared for use against tetanus contains a protective ANTIBODY against specific tetanus toxins. (When used against a toxin an antiserum is known as an antitoxin.)

One traditional method of producing tetanus antitoxin is to immunize an animal such as a horse with tetanus germs and then collect the antibodies from the horse's blood. The horse serum containing the protective antibodies is then injected into a human being who is at risk of developing tetanus. While at one time antiserum made from horses was quite commonly used against tetanus, the pharmaceutical industry today markets a tetanus antitoxin known as Humotet, derived almost exclusively from human beings.

ARTERIAL BLOOD GAS DETERMINATION The respiratory gases oxygen and carbon dioxide are normally found in the bloodstream. During a severe or prolonged asthma attack, important changes take place in the amounts of these gases in the body. In order to treat the asthmatic patient appropriately, a specimen of arterial blood is analysed for its blood gas concentration.

ASTHMA A condition characterized by reversible episodes of airway obstruction which range in severity from mild to life-threatening. Common symptoms include shortness of breath, chest tightness, coughing and wheezing. Children do not have to be allergic to have asthma, though they often are. Asthma can be broadly divided into three forms: allergic or extrinsic immunologic, nonallergic or intrinsic/autonomic, and mixed.

ATOPIC DERMATITIS A form of eczema, an allergic skin condition characterized by dry skin and a very itchy rash, commonly located on the cheeks, backs of the ears, elbows, wrists and backs of the knees.

ATOPY The state or condition of being allergic.

AUTOGENOUS Self-generated. In allergic medicine, most commonly used to describe a vaccine prepared from bacteria taken directly from a patient's body.

B CELLS One of two special types of white blood cells called lymphocytes produced in the bone marrow. *See* LYMPHOCYTE

BACTERIAL VACCINES Vaccines prepared from common bacteria. For example, streptococcus and staphylococcus vaccines are used in the treatment of so-called bacterial allergy.

At best the use of these vaccines must be considered controversial; and while we know that viral infections can play a definite role in triggering attacks of bronchial asthma, there is no sound evidence to prove that a person can become truly allergic to a specific bacteria. There is general agreement among experts that there is no use for bacterial vaccines in the treatment of allergic diseases.

BACTERIAL ALLERGY *See* BACTERIAL VACCINES

BASOPHIL A specific type of white blood cell which circulates freely throughout the bloodstream and is coated with IgE antibodies. When this cell is stimulated to release chemical MEDIATORS, an allergic reaction is set in motion. *See* MEDIATOR

BETA-ADRENERGIC AGENT *See* BRONCHODILATOR

BLOOD GASES Gases, such as oxygen and carbon dioxide, in constant circulation throughout the bloodstream. During a severe asthma attack insufficient amounts of oxygen reach the blood and increased levels of carbon dioxide accumulate.

BRONCHIAL CHALLENGE TEST Inhaling an aerosolized spray containing an ALLERGEN suspected of causing asthma. This procedure should be done under the direct supervision of a doctor, in a laboratory. The test can also be done using the drugs histamine or methacholine.

BRONCHODILATOR DRUG A drug that causes the bronchial tubes to relax and dilate, commonly used in the treatment of bronchial asthma, some forms of chronic bronchitis, and occasionally in adults suffering from emphysema. The two main types of bronchodilator drugs are methylxanthines such as THEOPHYLLINE and BETA-ADRENERGIC AGENTS such as salbutamol.

BRONCHOSPASM Constricting or narrowing of the bronchial air passageways that causes wheezing.

CHALLENGE TESTING *See* BRONCHIAL CHALLENGE TEST, NASAL CHALLENGE TEST, ORAL CHALLENGE TEST

CLINICAL ECOLOGY A controversial new area of medical practice in which a variety of vague, fairly common symptoms not generally felt to be allergic are attributed to an undiagnosed and unrecognized allergy. A number of the diagnostic and therapeutic procedures used by clinical ecologists have been found to be both unreliable and ineffective. There is at present no valid scientific evidence supporting the medical claims of this 'speciality' for many of its methods of diagnosis and treatment.

CONTACT DERMATITIS An allergic rash that appears after exposure to a plant, chemical or metallic object to which a person has become sensitized. Inflammation is always localized in the area of specific contact. Common examples include primula, skin reactions to cosmetics or detergents and sensitivity to the nickel found in jewellery.

CORTICOSTEROIDS A group of naturally occurring hormones and commercially prepared agents which are powerful anti-inflammatory and anti-allergic drugs. Cortisone, produced naturally by the adrenal glands and manufactured commercially by pharmaceutical companies, is the best known of this rather large family. Many side effects are associated with them, one of the most common being weight gain. Use of corticosteroids must *always* be closely supervised by a doctor.

CYTOTOXIC TESTING An unproven diagnostic test used for evaluating food allergies, which does *not* work. The US Food and Drug Administration has labelled this procedure 'unreliable as a diagnostic test'.

DANDERS The dead superficial layers of skin that flake off an animal, producing allergic symptoms in a sensitized person.

DECONGESTANTS Drugs used mainly for the control of nasal symptoms associated with the common cold, allergic rhinitis (hay fever) and vasomotor rhinitis. Both spray and drop forms should never be taken for more than five days in a row; if used for longer periods they may not only lose their effectiveness but will actually cause nasal congestion.

DERMATOGRAPHISM A congenital condition in which the skin has a high degree of irritability. A raised wheal and redness appear on the skin when it is stroked or rubbed with a blunt object. Because of this nonspecific response pattern, a child with dermatographism is not a satisfactory candidate for direct skin tests (scratch or prick/puncture). *See* RAST TEST

DESENSITIZATION *See* IMMUNOTHERAPY

DIRECT SKIN TEST The simplest and most sensitive method to detect the presence of allergic IgE ANTIBODIES. *See* INTRADERMAL TEST, PRICK/PUNCTURE TEST, SCRATCH TEST

DUST MITES Microscopic insects that live mainly in bed linen and are thought by some investigators to be the main allergen found in dust.

ECZEMA A condition of the skin characterized by a rash that is extremely itchy, scaly and dry. *See* ATOPIC DERMATITIS, CONTACT DERMATITIS

ECZEMATOUS Characteristic of a condition of ECZEMA.

ELIMINATION DIET A procedure whereby a certain food is eliminated from a patient's diet for a trial period and the patient's reaction observed. If the symptoms disappear, the food is reintroduced to see if the symptoms return. This procedure must be repeated twice before a definite relationship is proved between the specific food and the allergy symptom.

EMPHYSEMA A chronic lung disease, limited almost exclusively to adults, that causes destruction of the ALVEOLI. Rarely, if ever, is there any relationship between asthma and emphysema. Damage to the lungs in emphysema is permanent and the changes are irreversible.

ENVIRONMENTAL CONTROL With IMMUNOTHERAPY and pharmacotherapy, one of the three major methods of managing allergic conditions.

EOSINOPHIL A type of white blood cell of which allergic patients usually show an increased number in their bloodstream, determined by a differential white blood cell count.

ERYTHROCYTE SEDIMENTATION RATE (ESR) A blood test, taken by VENIPUNCTURE, which indicates whether an inflammation (infection) is present somewhere within a patient's body. If the ESR value is positive, then other more specific diagnostic tests must be performed.

EXERCISE-INDUCED ASTHMA (EIA) A condition in which wheezing occurs after a period of strenuous physical activity; most common during the colder months of the year, especially following outdoor exertion, it occurs in 70 to 80 per cent of all asthma patients.

FBC Full blood count, a blood test used to check the number of red blood cells, white blood cells and amount of haemoglobin in a patient's body and to study specific types of circulating white blood cells (a differential count) to determine the presence of infection, anaemia or allergy.

FUNGI *See* MOULDS

GASTROOESOPHAGEAL REFLUX REFLEX (GER) A condition that occurs due to an improperly functioning gastro-oesophageal sphincter muscle, which permits the backup of stomach fluids into the oesophagus. Associated with recurrent cough and wheezing in infancy, a number of tests exist to diagnose it. These include X-ray studies, barium swallow, checking the acid level of the oesophagus fluid (pH monitoring), and pressure studies (manometry). Treatment involves thickened feedings, propping the infant up in an upright position after meals, and possibly surgery to repair the oesophageal sphincter, if medical treatment fails.

GENERALIZED ALLERGIC REACTION A reaction involving several organ systems at once. May involve the lungs (wheezing), the skin (hives), the nose and eyes (sneezing and weeping), and the cardio-vascular system (rapid heartbeat, drop in blood pressure). *See* ANAPHYLAXIS

HAY FEVER A common term for a pattern of symptoms that occur during the pollinating seasons of trees, grasses and weeds, and which is medically known as SEASONAL RHINITIS. Symptoms may include a runny nose, sneezing, streaming, itchy eyes, nasal congestion, fatigue and irritability. There is no fever involved with hay fever, nor is it caused by hay.

HISTAMINE The cause of the itching, runny nose, streaming eyes and swelling typically associated with hay fever and eczema. *See* MEDIATOR

HIVES *See* URTICARIA

HOUSE DUST Dust composed of the breakdown products of organic fibres such as wool and cotton as well as animal danders, insect residues, bacteria, food substances, mould spores and so on. *See* DUST MITES

HYMENOPTERA An order of insects responsible for the majority of allergic sting reactions. Members include bees, wasps and hornets.

HYPERSENSITIVITY A state of the immune system in which harmful symptoms are produced in the individual, as opposed to the normally beneficial responses of the system. There are four major types of hypersensitivity response: ANAPHYLACTIC, cytotoxic, immune complex mediated and cell mediated or delayed.

HYPOALLERGENIC A term referring to substances which have a very low potential to sensitize people or to cause an allergic reaction.

HYPOSENSITIZATION *See* IMMUNOTHERAPY.

IMMEDIATE HYPERSENSITIVITY An allergic reaction involving the IgE class of immunoglobulin proteins, also referred to as anaphylactic hypersensitivity. Examples include allergic rhinitis, penicillin allergy, allergic asthma and anaphylactic shock.

IMMUNE SYSTEM The physiological system that guards and protects the body against bacteria, viruses, cancer cells, chemicals and, under certain unusual conditions, one's own organs. The immune system includes the thymus gland, the bone marrow, the lymph nodes (glands), the spleen and specialized lymph tissues in the intestinal tract. A number of different types of cells play a crucial role in this system. These include white blood cells calls LYMPHO-CYTES, eosinophils, and monocyte-macrophages. Without a properly functioning immune system, humans could not survive.

IMMUNOGLOBULINS Special type of protein produced by the body. There are five classes of immunoglobulins (Ig), designated IgM, IgA, IgD, IgG and IgE. The IgM, IgA and IgG classes are responsible for protecting the body against invasion by viruses and bacteria. The function of IgD is still unclear. IgE antibodies are involved primarily with allergic reactions.

The various immunoglobulins are produced by a special type of lymphocyte (a white blood cell) called a plasma cell.

IMMUNOTHERAPY A form of allergy treatment commonly referred to as 'desensitization', or hyposensitization. Treatment consists of increasing a patient's tolerance to an allergic substance by means of a graduated programme of injections that contain ever-increasing doses of the allergen. The average length of treatment can be anywhere from two to four years. When successful, immunotherapy will reduce the intensity and duration of clinical allergic symptoms, though it will not necessarily eliminate them completely. Recommended for allergic rhinitis, severe insect sting sensitivity and allergic asthma. This is no longer used because of the danger of fatal anaphylaxis, but it is hoped that some limited use may be made of it in the future.

INTRADERMAL TEST The most sensitive form of direct skin test available, in which a small amount of allergen is injected by a needle or syringe into the superficial layers of the skin.

IN VITRO TEST A test done in the laboratory.

IN VIVO TEST A test done directly on the patient.

KAPOK A fibre derived from the kapok tree, commonly used as a filler for decorative pillows and a stuffing for upholstered furniture. It is a common allergen.

LACTOSE INTOLERANCE A condition arising from the absence of an enzyme called lactase in the small intestine and generally characterized by chronic diarrhoea. Often seen in infants, its symptoms begin shortly after the introduction of either human or cow's milk to the diet and tend to clear up immediately if a nonmilk formula such as a soybean preparation is substituted. Lactose intolerance is usually a lifelong condition, and sufferers must make all efforts to avoid all sources of milk such as milk, cheese, cream and so on. This is not an allergic condition but rather an enzyme deficiency disease.

LUNG FUNCTION TEST *See* PULMONARY FUNCTION TEST

LYMPHOCYTE A type of white blood cell that plays an important role in the immune process. In one of its specialized forms, as a plasma cell it is responsible for producing ANTIBODIES. Classified into two groups: the T cell lymphocyte that originates in the thymus gland and the B cell lymphocyte that comes from bone marrow. A complicated relationship exists between the B and T lymphocytes, as they work together in many types of immune responses.

MAST CELL A cell found in body tissues, coated with IgE antibodies in allergic individuals. When these antibodies react with their specific antigens, an allergic reaction takes place, the end result being the release of a number of chemical MEDIATORS (such as HISTAMINE or SRS-A) with the consequent development of allergic symptoms.

MEDIATOR A chemical compound released from the basophil and mast cells during an allergic reaction. Sneezing, weeping, a watery, drippy nose and wheezing are the most typical allergic symptoms caused by the various chemical mediators. *See* HISTAMINE, SRS-A

MOULDS Plants that do not possess chlorophyll and which therefore depend on outside sources of nourishment. Over 75,000 different varieties have been identified, many of which may cause allergic symptoms. *See* SPORES

MUCUS The viscous fluid secreted by the mucus glands to moisten and protect the MUCOUS MEMBRANES. Mucus varies in consistency from a thin, watery secretion to a thick, yellow-green discharge. Mucus-secreting glands line the respiratory tract from the nose to the smallest airways of the lungs.

MUCOUS MEMBRANES The linings of the mouth, throat, nose and respiratory system.

NASAL CHALLENGE TEST This is a test in which a suspension containing a suspected ALLERGEN is sprayed into the nose in order to determine if the person is allergic. The procedure should always be done in a laboratory, supervised by a doctor.

NASAL POLYPS Round, soft, jellylike masses found in the sinuses and nasal passageways. Most commonly clear to whitish in colour, they may grow individually or in grape-like clusters. In childhood they are most commonly associated with cystic fibrosis. While severely allergic children can under certain conditions develop polyps, they are more commonly found in adults. Treatment for polyps requires the use of topical cortisone sprays as a shrinking agent. If this measure fails, surgical removal is often the only alternative; unfortunately there is a high rate of regrowth of surgically removed polyps.

ORAL CHALLENGE TEST Eating a food containing a suspected ALLERGEN to determine if an allergy is present; always done under the direct supervision of a doctor.

OTITIS MEDIA An inflammation of the middle ear especially common in young children.

PATCH TEST A method used to identify substances responsible for causing allergic responses, specially CONTACT DERMATITIS. The suspected material is placed on a small area of the skin, usually on the arm or back, and covered with an adhesive patch. After forty-eight hours the test site is checked. The presence of an itchy, blistery area is considered to be a positive response, indicating that the person is allergic to the test substance.

PENICILLIN ALLERGY One of the most common types of drug allergy, the symptoms of which can range from a mild skin rash to a life-threatening, generalized, ANAPHYLACTIC response. A method of testing for this allergy exists but can identify a person who is allergic to penicillin only after the individual has displayed some symptoms.

POLLEN A grain containing the male reproductive portion of trees, grasses and weeds. Microscopically small, it is carried long distances by the wind. Allergy to this pollen is responsible for the symptoms of such conditions as allergic rhinitis and asthma.

PRICK TEST A form of direct skin test in which a drop of allergen is placed on the arm or back and the point of a needle is used to puncture the skin so that the allergen is able to react with the tissue mast cells.

PROVOCATIVE TESTING A procedure exposing patients to a specific allergen to determine if they are allergic to it. *See* BRONCHIAL CHALLENGE TEST, NASAL CHALLENGE TEST, ORAL CHALLENGE TEST

PRURITIS The medical term for itching.

PULMONARY FUNCTION TEST A test designed to obtain specific information indicating how efficiently a patient's lungs are operating.

RAST TEST (RADIOALLERGOSORBENT TEST) An in vitro method of allergy testing in which blood serum is examined and analysed. Though generally reliable, it is less sensitive than certain forms of direct skin testing such as the INTRADERMAL TEST. It is also expensive and requires a good deal of time before the results are known. When direct skin tests cannot be performed, the RAST test is an acceptable alternative.

REAGINIC ANTIBODIES A term that refers to allergic antibodies of the IgE class of IMMUNOGLOBULINS.

REBOUND PHENOMENON A response to a medicine in which clinical symptoms worsen after the medication is discontinued.

RHINITIS A nasal condition characterized by sneezing, nasal congestion and an increase in nasal discharge. Rhinitis can occur on a seasonal basis (when it is known as hay fever or rose fever) or it may be year-round, as in perennial allergic rhinitis. *See* VASOMOTOR RHINITIS.

RHINITIS MEDICAMENTOSA A condition that develops owing to prolonged use of vasoconstrictor nose drops or sprays.

RINKEL METHOD A controversial and unproven technique of immunotherapy using a graduated testing schedule; the purpose of this method is to determine both the appropriate starting dose and the so-called endpoint of therapy. Controlled studies have proved, however, that the endpoint dose is simply too low to produce a maximal response.

SCRATCH TEST A procedure administered by placing a drop of ALLERGEN on the arm or back. A superficial scratch is made over the test site with the tip of a needle so that the allergen is absorbed directly into the skin.

SENSITIZED Any person who has been exposed to an antigen (a foreign substance) that has stimulated the immune system to produce specific antibodies has become sensitized. For example, the hay-fever sufferer has been sensitized to pollen.

SERUM The clear, yellowish liquid portion of the blood that remains

after a clot has formed and the white and red blood cells have
settled out.

SHOCK ORGAN The part of the body that is the site of an allergic
reaction. The shock organ for allergic rhinitis is the nose; for
bronchial asthma it is the lungs.

SODIUM CROMOGLYCATE The generic name for a drug used to treat
asthma (in the form of Intal), allergic rhinitis (as Rynacrom) and
allergic conjunctivitis (as Opticrom). Unlike BRONCHODILATOR
DRUGS, which actively dilate the bronchial airways during an
asthma attack, sodium cromoglycate has the ability to prevent the
symptoms of asthma from developing. Sodium cromoglycate has
an extremely low incidence of side effects, which makes it
especially safe for children.

SRS-A An abbreviation for slow-reacting substance of anaphylaxis,
a powerful bronchoconstrictor MEDIATOR that is probably responsible for the severe prolonged bronchospasm which occurs during
an asthma attack. Now known as leukotrienes.

STATUS ASTHMATICUS A term describing an asthma attack so severe
that it does not respond to oral and inhaled BRONCHODILATOR
DRUGS. Patients who fail to respond to two or three injections of
ADRENALINE given at twenty-to-thirty-minute intervals are in status
asthmaticus and will require hospitalization for more intensive
treatment, which will usually include the administration of intravenous fluids, oxygen and cortisone.

STEROIDS *See* CORTICOSTEROIDS

SPORES Parts of the mould plant which contain the reproductive
system. Microscopic, they float in the air and are found in
profusion during spring, summer and early autumn; a primary
allergen for many allergy sufferers.

THEOPHYLLINE One of the xanthine group of BRONCHODILATOR DRUGS.
Is less used than it used to be, having been supplanted to a large
extent by the beta-adrenergic drugs.

TYMPANOMETRY A sensitive procedure used to check for abnormalities of the tympanic membrane/middle-ear/eustachian tube system and to evaluate middle ear function; it is painless and can be done in a surgery with children as young as seven months.

URTICARIA A localized swelling in the superficial layers of the skin, commonly known as hives or nettle rash. The typical rash consists of red or white raised lesions surrounded by a reddish border; it can be recognized most directly by its severe, persistent itching. *See* ANGIOEDEMA.

VASOMOTOR RHINITIS A nasal condition characterized by symptoms which closely mimic those of HAY FEVER: nasal congestion, sneezing and (occasionally) a year-round runny nose; it occurs as a result of a nonspecific irritative response to a variety of *nonallergic* stimuli and is localized to the mucous membranes of the nose. This condition tends to become chronic, and treatment is geared towards controlling symptoms; so far no permanent cure exists.

VENOMS *See* HYMENOPTERA

WHEEZE The typical rattling, whistling, breathing sounds an asthmatic child makes when exhaling, primarily owing to the narrowing of the breathing tubes and the accumulation of thick mucus secretions within the air passageways.

Index